CANCER
PREVENTION

CANCER PREVENTION
Strategies in the Workplace

Edited by

Charles E. Becker
and
Molly Joel Coye

University of California Medical Center
and San Francisco General Hospital

⬤ HEMISPHERE PUBLISHING CORPORATION, Washington
A subsidiary of Harper & Row, Publishers, Inc.

Cambridge   New York   Philadelphia   San Francisco
London   Mexico City   São Paulo   Singapore   Sydney

CANCER PREVENTION: Strategies in the Workplace

1 2 3 4 5 6 7 8 9 0   B R B R   8 9 8 7 6

Library of Congress Cataloging-in-Publication Data
Main entry under title:

Cancer prevention.

  Based on the Second Annual Occupational Cancer
Conference in San Francisco in 1984: sponsored by the
University of California School of Medicine and others.
  Includes bibliographies and index.
  1. Cancer—Prevention—Congresses. 2. Occupational
diseases—Prevention—Congresses. 3. Carcinogens—
Congresses. I. Becker, Charles Earl, date.
II. Coye, Molly. III. Occupational Cancer Conference
(2nd : 1984 : San Francisco, Calif.) IV. University
of California, San Francisco. School of Medicine.
[DNLM: 1. Carcinogens—congresses. 2. Neoplasms—
prevention & control—United States—congresses.
3. Occupational Diseases—prevention & control—United
States—congresses.   QZ 200 C215367 1984]
RC268.C366   1986   362.1'9699'4   86-1983
ISBN 0-89116-441-3

Contents

Contributors

Olav Axelson, M.D.
Department of Occupational
  Medicine
University Hospital
S-581 85 Linkoping, Sweden

Charles E. Becker, M.D.
Division of Occupational and
  Environmental Health
Department of Medicine
University of California, San
  Francisco
San Francisco General Hospital
San Francisco, CA 94110

Neal L. Benowitz, M.D.
Department of Medicine
University of California, San
  Francisco
San Francisco General Hospital
San Francisco, CA 94110

Thomas D. Boyer, M.D.
Department of Medicine
University of California, San
  Francisco
Veterans Administration
  Medical Center
San Francisco, CA 94121

Ed Cadman, M.D.
Department of Medicine
University of California, San
  Francisco
San Francisco, CA 94143

James E. Cone, M.D., M.P.H.
Occupational Health Clinic
University of California, San
  Francisco
San Francisco General Hospital
San Francisco, CA 94110

Molly Joel Coye, M.D.
Department of Medicine
University of California, San
  Francisco
San Francisco General Hospital
San Francisco, CA 94110

Lois Swirsky Gold, Ph.D.
Biology and Medicine Division
Lawrence Berkeley Laboratory
Berkeley, CA 94720

Lennart Hardell, M.D.
Department of Oncology
University Hospital
S-901 85 Umea, Sweden

Kim Hooper, Ph.D.
Epidemiologic Studies
Department of Health Services
State of California
Berkeley, CA 94704

Joseph LaDou, M.D.
Division of Occupational and
  Environmental Medicine
Department of Medicine
University of California, San
  Francisco
San Francisco, CA 94143

C. G. Toby Mathias, M.D.
Department of Dermatology
University of California, San
  Francisco
San Francisco General Hospital
San Francisco, CA 94110

Stephen McCurdy, M.D.,
  M.P.H.
Department of Internal
  Medicine
University of California, Davis
Davis, CA 95616

John Osterloh, M.D.
Department of Medicine
University of California, San
  Francisco
San Francisco General Hospital
San Francisco, CA 94110

Luci A. Power, M.S.
Pharmaceutical Services
University of California, San
  Francisco Hospitals and
  Clinics
San Francisco, CA 94143

Jon Rosenberg, M.D.
Department of Medicine
University of California, San
  Francisco
San Francisco General Hospital
San Francisco, CA 94110

Marc Schenker, M.D., M.P.H.
Department of Internal
  Medicine
University of California, Davis
Davis, CA 95616

Allan H. Smith
Northern California
  Occupational Health Center
University of California,
  Berkeley
Berkeley, CA 94720

Martyn T. Smith
Department of Biomedical and
  Environmental Health
  Sciences
School of Public Health
University of California,
  Berkeley
Berkeley, CA 94720

Joseph W. Sullivan
Northern California
  Occupational Health Center
University of California,
  Berkeley
Berkeley, CA 94720

Preface

Great strides have been made in identifying subtle changes in cells exposed to cancer-causing agents. However, our understanding of the significance of these subtle changes is still incomplete. Chemicals posing a risk to society are present in food, drinking water, air, and the workplace. As a result, great public pressure is now being applied to scientists for conclusive information concerning the risk to the public from cancer-causing materials. Because we do not understand fully the mechanisms of normal cell function, it has been difficult for scientists to quantitatively assess the risk of cancer. The human working population is so heterogeneous that estimates of "safe" levels of exposure to most chemicals do not exist. As these uncertainties become apparent, community and worker right-to-know legislation places demands on the scientific community to devise valid strategies to safeguard the public. Despite differences in scientific opinion, one factor is evident: Occupational exposures that contribute to cancer are, by definition, caused by society, and therefore can be prevented.

Because of the growing need to make the public and scientific community more aware of the methods for preventing occupational cancer, the University of California School of Medicine in conjunction with the Northern California Occupational Health Center, the National Institutes of Occupational Safety and Health, and the American Cancer Society sponsored the Second Annual Occupational Cancer Conference in San Francisco in late 1984. Because of the enthusiasm and interest of the participants at this conference, 13 of these presentations are prepared for this text.

It was evident to all present at the conference that even though it is extraordinarily difficult to define "safe" levels of human exposure to any suspected carcinogen, there is the need to bring together existing scientific information and to promote further research to assist in our understanding of the basic mechanism of cancer. While this research process advances methods of identifying cancer-causing agents, strategies for preventing their exposure in the workplace must continue to be practiced. The workplace provides a valuable setting for estimating the incidence of cancer and a model for preventive strategy to protect workers and society.

Charles E. Becker

Molly Joel Coye

CANCER PREVENTION

1

Occupational Cancer:
Past and Present

CHARLES E. BECKER and MOLLY JOEL COYE

INTRODUCTION

In the last ten years great strides have been made in precisely identifying and quantitating subtle perturbations of cells when exposed to suspected chemical agents; yet our ability to understand the significance of these changes is still deficient. Public pressure for regulatory preventive action results in demands on scientists for conclusive statements regarding the identification of carcinogenic materials or the explanation of subtle changes in cell systems. Recent public attention directed towards the presence of potentially carcinogenic materials in food stuffs and in drinking water supplies are dramatic examples of the public and scientific pressure which can be generated. Scientific consultants and legislators are now forced to make important decisions with limited scientific information.

Cancer kills approximately 430,000 individuals in the United States annually (1). The American Cancer Society estimates that some form of cancer will develop in one-fourth of the American population. Cancer is the second leading cause of death and the second leading cause of lost years of potential life in this country. Recent attention has focused on behavioral factors such as cigarette smoking, alcohol, drug abuse and sexual activity that contribute to cancer prevalence. In evaluating the extent to which a given cancer has an occupational etiology, scientists have been slow to appreciate the risk of previous occupational exposures to cancer.

Evidence for a relationship between occupational exposures and cancer comes primarily from epidemiological studies and toxicological studies in animals. Although general agreement exists concerning the overall incidence of cancer, considerable controversy surrounds the proportion of cancers that can be attributed solely to occupational exposures. Since the mechanism of carcinogenesis is still not fully appreciated, different experimental models and observational epidemiological studies have tended to provide the best information. Yet, several characteristics of occupationally-related cancers contribute to the difficulty in making these estimates. Finding a specific cohort with a unique exposure is often extraordinarily difficult because industrial agents are not confined solely to the workplace but pollute the local environment as well. The range of potential exposures is also difficult to encompass in a study: there are well over 6 million chemicals in the computerized registry of the chemical abstract services of the American Chemical Society, with approximately 500 new chemicals per year proposed for toxicological evaluation. Since there are now some 60 to 70,000 chemicals in common use, of which less than 10 percent have been tested adequately for carcinogenicity in the experimental animals, the limitations of data available at present are marked (2).

Cancers that are related to occupation are often characterized by a long latency. Tumors may develop many years after exposure, making it difficult to characterize and quantitate risk factors. In addition, individuals with cancer may have been exposed to several different carcinogens which interact with one another. Cigarette smoking, alcohol consumption and dietary factors may interact with occupational factors, making scientific assessment more difficult. Information may also be lacking on the character and the duration of the exposure, making dose response relationships difficult to assess.

The documentation of the specific site and type of cancer has also been fraught with difficulty. Errors in pathological and clinical diagnoses of cancer are common. American citizens have been notoriously resistant to structuring a nation-wide tracking system for vital statistics which would allow for meaningful methods of obtaining occupational histories. In only a few states is information collected on work histories of cancer victims to provide sufficient data for analysis. The identification of possible occupational etiologies for cancer have been achieved for malignant diseases which are rare, such as mesothelioma (asbestos exposure) and angiosarcoma of the liver (vinyl chloride exposure). However, significant differences in the rates of total cancer among small subgroups of workers may be overlooked because the baseline rates for overall cancer incidence are not detected in a large study population. Despite these drawbacks, the study of cancer mortality from workplace exposures has proven to be one of the most productive avenues of research in identifying causes of human cancer. Of all the agents or processes generally accepted as carcinogenic in humans, more have been identified in studies of occupation than from any other source. Currently there are approximately 18 agents or processes which have been listed by the International Agency for Research on Cancer as causally associated with cancers in humans. In terms of immediate impact on mortality, occupational exposure is one of the most important specific factors quantitatively identified as causative of human cancer in the United States, with the most important exposure, asbestos, associated with more than 8,500 projected deaths annually (3).

It is important to emphasize that most occupational carcinogens were first identified by alert physicians or pathologists who had a high clinical index of suspicion for these etiologies. As the human life span continues to increase with improved health care delivery, it is likely that the volume and diversity of chemicals manufactured in this country will affect the future incidence of cancer produced. It is for these reasons that improved understanding of the mechanism of cancer causation, improved surveillance techniques and better understanding of risk assessment procedures will be applied to this growing field. The need for cancer prevention is best illustrated by the estimates that approximately 1.2 million people each year develop cancer. Nearly half of these will be cured by surgical resection of the tumor before metastasis occurs. Yet, nearly 600,000 individuals will have disseminated cancer with only 50,000 being cured by chemotherapy or radiation. It is clear from this information that the treatment of cancer is only helpful for approximately half of all the people with the disease. Thus, the most cost effective approach is to prevent cancer from developing. Since by definition cancer caused by an occupational agent is "man-caused," they are by definition preventable. Substitutions of carcinogenic chemicals, enforcement of protective standards for exposure, design and application of engineering controls and use of personal protective equipment by exposed workers all are useful prevention strategies.

EPIDEMIOLOGY

The relationship of human exposure to a potentially
carcinogenic material is studied by three methods:
epidemiological studies, long-term animal studies and
short-term tests in vitro. Epidemiology has contributed
substantially to the knowledge about the origins of
human cancer and provides the foundation for measures
designed to prevent cancer. The major strength of
epidemiological studies is the focus on human
populations, avoiding extrapolations from whole animal
or short-term in vitro screening methods.
Epidemiological studies of cancer prevalence throughout
the world suggest that for total cancer the variation
may be as much as three-fold, whereas the range of rates
for certain anatomical sites may vary one-hundred-fold.
Although some of this variation in cancer prevalence may
have a genetic basis, a major role for occupational
factors has clearly been demonstrated. Although we must
learn much more about the factors responsible for
geographic and temporal variations of cancer incidence
in the general population, epidemiological studies tend
to confirm that cancer results from the combined effects
of multiple exposures and unique susceptibility states.

Epidemiology studies currently suggest that the
multistage models for cancer production in which
different risk factors accelerate the transition rates
at various stages of carcinogenesis is most plausible.
Tobacco, solar radiation, ionizing radiation, infectious
agents and medications have all been identified
epidemiologically with accelerated risks of cancer.
Epidemiology has also suggested that genetic factors
appear to contribute to the high rates of some
malignancies, especially those of the nasopharynx, gall
bladder and skin. Epidemiology has not been able to
fully study familial susceptibility compared to
environmental factors such as smoking and lung cancer or
sunlight and skin cancer. Using carefully performed case
control methods or cohort analyses, major progress has
occurred. However, epidemiology studies have gained
limited acceptance in establishing causal relationships
because it has been difficult to exclude bias and
confounding exposures and dose response relationships
have often been lacking. In addition, with greater
awareness of the occupational factors contributing to
cancer there has been an overall reduction in exposures
in industry, fortunately providing fewer workers with
high exposures for easy study.

The most important limiting features of epidemiology are
the inability to obtain good occupational information
and exposure data. It has been extraordinarily difficult
to study existing data information linking deaths or
cancer production with taxation systems, the Census

Bureau or the Social Security Administration. Using population-based tumor registries to identify occupational groups at high risk for developing cancer has become popular (4). It is evident from such studies that negative or statistically non-significant findings are of limited value, due to short observational periods and small sample sizes. However, record linkage for high risk populations has proved to be an effective means of identifying occupational causes for cancer, especially specific cancer sites.

OCCUPATIONAL CANCER RISK ASSESSMENT

Methods of establishing risk assessment have been suggested using many different animal species and over 130 short-term in vivo methods for detecting chemicals which induce cell changes. Risk assessment is extraordinarily risky. There are so many components in a scientific assessment of occupational cancer risk that the choice among scientific interpretations cannot be guided by science alone - because there is no general agreement on the methods or models which should be used. Without full knowledge about the mechanisms of cancer causation, the choice between various risk assessment models provokes major controversy. The rapid pace of scientific growth in this area has made carcinogen risk assessment even more fraught with controversy. Several States have attempted to draft guidelines to clarify internal procedures on which risk assessment can be performed, and the Office of Science and Technology has recently summarized in the Federal Registry the scientific basis for many assumptions in many of these methods (5). It is evident from this scientific review as well as the documents generated by several states that short term tests, when properly used and validated, can provide strong indications of potential carcinogenicity. However, based upon our current limited knowledge of the mechanism of cancer induction, it appears that there will be some classes of potential carcinogens that are not detected by the currently available short term methods. The utilization of long term animal studies for quantitative occupational human risk assessment has focused attention on the scientific uncertainties involved in the relationship of animal to human cancer risk. Nonetheless, animal studies with all of their limitations are currently one of the best ways of predicting effects in humans when epidemiological studies are unavailable.

It is evident that many more agents will be identified as carcinogenic by animals than by short term tests or epidemiology. There are currently approximately 86 compounds used in occupational settings which are

carcinogenic in animals. Only 18 agents have sufficient
evidence of carcinogenicity in humans; 33 are
considered probable carcinogens in humans (6).
Fortunately, the concordance between human and animal
studies is probably acceptable. Yet animal studies have
substantial limitations. A standard bioassay of two
exposures in males and females with two different
species of 60 animals each involving 500 rodents will
cost some $500,000. Thus a standard bioassay is a major
financial and scientific undertaking. Nicholson (6)
estimates that the cost of tracing and follow-up on
epidemiological mortality study costs approximately $100
per person. Therefore, only cancer risks of the orders
of one in ten at a maximum tolerated dose can be
established definitively by bioassays. That risk
corresponds to a 10 to 100 fold risk. For agents with
less potency, exposures of much higher intensity are
required far more than that experienced by humans. Thus,
lower human exposure circumstances must be evaluated
using other appropriate extrapolation models. Yet many
carcinogenic agents may not be capable of identification
either by animal bioassays or studies of human
populations because of study limitations (6).

MECHANISM OF CANCER PRODUCTION

It is evident that chemicals used in the workplace can
cause cancer in humans and animals. Some chemical
carcinogens act directly on cell populations whereas
others must be metabolized to produce carcinogens.
Because of the wide variety of carcinogen structures and
modifications that are necessary, a simple explanation
for chemical carcinogen seems unlikely. We simply do not
know whether a single cell or a single group of cells
are transformed to cause cancer. It is also possible
that normal cells may carry the seeds of transformation
to cancer in the form of cancer genes known as
oncogenes. It is evident that our increased
understanding of the biology of cancer has made it more
difficult to form a simple explanation for cancer
production. Smuckler has reviewed in detail chemicals
and their ability to cause cancer (7). Despite an
increasing ability to measure cellular components and
chemicals in the environment our knowledge about the
meaning of these chemical changes has not kept pace with
our ability to identify them. Because we cannot explain
the mechanism for cancer formation or the role of
chemicals in the process, we must act with insufficient
information to make important decisions for individuals
and society. Several panels (8) have also struggled with
chemical carcinogenesis. These studies have suggested
that chemical carcinogenesis evaluation must take into
account _in vitro_ tests, metabolism studies and biometric

analyses as well as many other variables. Any one method
alone cannot produce a reliable estimate of the
chemical's cancer risk to man. Taken together, however,
these studies can provide a high level of confidence in
predicting human cancer. Because chemical carcinogenesis
is a rapidly moving field and with massive quantities of
data being accumulated, it is essential that scientific
information be reviewed often and scientific advances
fully appreciated. The interdisciplinary panel on
carcinogenicity (8) concluded "because of the strengths
and weakness of the data to be evaluated in the
assessment of human risk and the complexity of the
problem, case by case analysis is most appropriate." To
assist in this work Ames and his colleagues have
developed a generally accepted format for the numerical
description of carcinogenic potency of particular
chemicals in a particular strain of animals. This
"Carcinogenic Potency Database" which includes results
of 3000 longterm and chronic experiments of 770 test
compounds may permit comparison of carcinogenic potency.
It also may provide quantitative information about
negative tests. This impressive work covers a
carcinognic potency range over 10 million fold (9, 10).

CONCLUSION

The search for the methods of preventing occupational
cancer has stimulated a new cohort of scientific
investigators and has advanced our basic understanding
of cell function. Until we fully understand the
mechanism of cancer production, it will be impossible to
estimate "safe" levels of human exposures. The human
population is not an inbred strain. Cancer risk
assessment provides a perplexing array of scientific
problems. If we have learned anything from over the past
200 years since the description of scrotal cancer in
chimney sweeps, it has been that cancer production in
the workplace is extraordinarily complicated. Community
and worker right to know legislation will continue to
place pressure upon scientists to communicate to
citizens scientific uncertainties. Establishing risks of
cancer must involve thoughtfull communication so as to
make risks if present acceptable and voluntary. While
differences of scientific opinion will definitely exist,
it is evident that occupational exposures that
contribute to cancer are clearly preventable.

In order to enhance the awareness and timeliness of new
information concerning preventive methods for
occupational cancer, the University of California School
of Medicine, in conjunction with the Northern California
Occupational Health Center, the National Institutes of
Occupational Safety and Health and the American Cancer
Society, sponsored the Second Annual Recent Advances in

Occupational Cancer Conference on December 7th and 8th,
1984 in San Francisco, California. A portion of the
first conference was published after enthusiastic
support by conference participants (11). This text
covers 13 presentations from this conference. The key
note address by Edwin C. Cadmen stresses the basic
biology of cancer and emphasizes that cancer is a
preventable disease. Special controversial topics are
also addressed, such as Dr. Neal Benowitz's review of
the importance of side stream smoke in the etiology of
and lung cancer, Lenard Hardell's review of phenoxy
herbicides and other pesticides in the etiology of
cancer, Lucy Powers' review of the handling of
oncological agents, and Thomas Boyer's review of
environmental agents in the causation of hepatic
malignancy. Specialized industries are also addressed
at this conference: Marc Schenker reviews solvents and
pesticides in the etiology of cancer in agriculture
workers; C.G. Toby Mathias reviews occupational skin
cancers; Joseph LaDou reviews low level asbestos
exposure in air and water supply; Jim Cone reviews PCB
risks in fires, accidents and printing and John
Osterloh reviews the carcinogenic potential of ethylene
dibromide, Jon Rosenberg reviews formaldehyde toxicity,
and Martyn T. Smith reviews collaborative work done by
R.E. Talcott on quinones as mutagens, carcinogens and
anticancer agents. Finally, Kim Hooper reviews
mechanisms of cancer production.

It was evident to all participants that there is
concern that focusing attention on life style matters
such as smoking, alcohol and diet may ignore the
importance of the workplace as a hazardous environment.
The primary means for preventing occupational cancer is
through eliminating exposures. Since it is
extraordinarily difficult to define a safe level of
human exposure to any suspected carcinogen there is a
critical need for more research to assist us in
prevening cancer associated with workplace exposure and
for policies to reduce occupational exposures while
this research is carried out.

REFERENCES

1. MMWR March 9, 1984, 33:9.

2. Schottenfeld D.: Chronic Disease in the Workplace:
   Cancer. Archives of Environ Hlth 39:(3) May and June,
   1984, pp. 150-157.

3. Nicholson WJ: Research Issues on Occupational and
   Environmental Cancer. Arch Environ Hlth 39(3):190-
   202, May and June, 1984.

4. Whorton D.M., Schulman J., Larson S.R., Stubbs, H.A. and Austin.: Feasibility of Identifying HIgh Risk Occupations through Tumor Registries. J Occup Med 25(9):657-660, Sept, 1983.

5. Federal Registry, Thursday, March 14, 1985, Part Two. Office of Science and Technology Policy "Chemical Carcinogens: A Review of the Science and Its Associated Principles." February, 1985.

6. Nicholson W.J.: Research Issues in Occupational and Environmental Cancer. Arch Environ Hlth 39(3): May & June, 1984.

7. Smuckler, E.A.: Chemicals. Cancer and Cancer Biology. West J Med 133(1):55-74, July, 1983.

8. Interdisciplinary panels on carcinogenicity. Criteria for Evidence of Chemical Carcinogenicity. Science 225:682-687, 1984.

9. Peto et al.: The TD 50: A Proposed General Convention for Numerical Description of the Carcinogenic Potency of Chemicals in Chronic Exposure Animal Experiments. Environ Hlth Persp 58:1-8, 1984.

10. Gold LS et al.: A Carcinogenic Potency Data Base of Standardized Results of Animal Bioassays. Environ Hlth Persp 68:9-319, 1984.

11. Becker C.E., Coye, M.J.: Recent Advances in Occupational Cancer. J Toxicol 22(3) 1984.

2

The Exposure-Potency Index (EPI): Ranking Carcinogenic Hazards of Volatile Industrial Chemicals

KIM HOOPER and LOIS SWIRSKY GOLD

SUMMARY

Employers, employees, and occupational health professionals
need a simple index to rank carcinogens according to their
potential danger at exposure levels which are commonly
encountered in workplaces. We describe such an index, the
Exposure-Potency Index (EPI). This simple proportion, dose
level (mg/kg body weight/day) to which workers are permitted
to be exposed/cancer-causing dose (mg/kg body weight/day) in
test animals, permits comparisons among carcinogens. We
have calculated this index for inhalation exposures to 1,3-
butadiene, 1,2-dibromo-3-chloropropane (DBCP), 1,2-
dibromoethane (EDB), ethylene oxide, formaldehyde, unleaded
gasoline vapors, methylene chloride, propylene oxide, and
trichloroethylene (TCE). The permitted worker exposure
levels have frequently been close to the levels which induce
tumors in laboratory animals. More recently, Permissible
Exposure Limits (PEL's) for some chemicals have been
markedly reduced, and this is reflected in lowered EPI
values. Combining EPI values with information on the
numbers of exposed workers provides a simple means of
identifying and ranking dangers to populations of workers.

INTRODUCTION

Those concerned with occupational health (e.g. employers,
employees, occupational health professionals, unions, and
regulatory agencies) need a way to rank the potential
dangers posed by occupational carcinogens at exposure levels
that are likely to be encountered in workplaces. At
present, 23 chemicals or groups of chemicals and 7
industrial processes have been causally associated with
cancer in humans, and nearly 200 have been evaluated by the

International Agency for Research on Cancer (IARC) as
carcinogenic to animals (IARC, 1985). Given the large
number of carcinogens and the variety of workplace
exposures, a simple method is needed to flag those agents
which may present greater risks.

THE EXPOSURE-POTENCY INDEX

One index of the potential danger faced by a worker exposed
to an occupational carcinogen would be the simple ratio
between the lifetime exposure (mg/kg body weight/day) the
worker receives and the lifetime dose level (mg/kg body
weight/day) that induces tumors in animals. Unfortunately,
exposure assessments of workplace chemicals are frequently
incomplete or uneven at best, so the actual average daily
dose levels that workers receive are not accurately known.
However, Permissible Exposure Limits (PEL's) have been set
by regulatory agencies for 400-500 chemicals. (Many of
these chemicals have not been tested for carcinogenicity.)
These occupational standards can be used as surrogates for
actual workplace exposure levels. The PEL is the maximum
allowable concentration of an airborne contaminant in
workplace air on a time-weighted average basis over an 8-
hour day and 40-hour week. Thus, the PEL should represent
the maximum dose a worker would receive over an 8-hour work
day.

Using the PEL as a surrogate for workplace exposure, we
estimate the Exposure-Potency Index (EPI) as

$$EPI = \frac{\text{permitted exposure level to worker (mg/kg/day)}}{\text{dose to induce tumors in animals (mg/kg/day)}} \times 100 \quad \quad 1)$$

In Equation 1, the numerator is the exposure level (mg/kg
body weight/day) which a worker is permitted to receive over
a working lifetime of 40 years, i.e. the Occupational
Effective Dose (OED). The denominator is the dose (mg/kg
body weight/day) that produces significant increases in
tumor incidence in test animals, i.e. the Cancer Effective
Dose (CED). The EPI expresses the exposure that workers are
permitted to receive as a percent of the dose that produced
a statistically significant increase in tumor incidence in
test animals. The larger the EPI value for a chemical, the
more concerned we are that permitted exposure levels may be
too high.

In present usage, "hazard" generally refers to the intrinsic
toxicity of a substance, and "risk" is estimated from the
results of both hazard and exposure assessments (OTA, 1985).

Thus, a cancer hazard index would rank an intrinsic property
of substances, e.g. carcinogenic potency, on an appropriate
dose scale (Meselson and Russell, 1977; Crouch and Wilson,
1979; Ames, et al, 1980; Gold, et al, 1984; and Peto, et al,
1984). The EPI couples potency with permissible exposure.

CANCER EFFECTIVE DOSE

The Cancer Effective Dose (CED) is defined as the lowest
chronic dose (mg/kg/day) of a chemical which produces
statistically significant (p<0.05) increases in neoplasms in
test animals, consistent with the author's evaluation of
carcinogenicity. CED values are calculated according to
Equation 2,

$$CED = \frac{(\text{exposure level in mg/M3})(\text{inhalation vol/day})}{(\text{body weight of test animal})} \quad 2)$$

using standard inhalation and body weights for rats and mice
and assuming 100% absorption (see Gold, et al., 1984). In
order to make comparisons among EPI values, CED values
should be standardized; in this paper, CED values have been
adjusted to approximate the dose that induces tumors in 50%
of the animals.

In chronic animal cancer bioassays, the dose may be
administered by oral, inhalation, injection, or dermal
routes. Inhalation is a preferred route of administration
for simulating workplace exposures to dusts, fumes and
volatile solvents. However, the oral route (gavage, diet,
or water) is most frequently used. CED values calculated
from ingestion bioassays can also be used to rank chemicals.

OCCUPATIONAL EFFECTIVE DOSE

The Occupational Effective Dose (OED) is defined as the
average lifetime daily dose a worker can legally receive by
inhaling airborne concentrations of a chemical at the PEL
for 5 days/week over a 40-year worklife. The OED is
calculated from Equation 2, using the PEL and standard
values for inhalation volume/day, body weight, and lifespan
for humans, and assuming 100% absorption.

EPI VALUES FROM INHALATION EXPOSURES

Inhalation is the major route of exposure for many
industrial chemicals (e.g. the carcinogenic solvents
benzene, trichloroethylene, and methylene chloride).
Because of this, the major thrust of occupational standards
has been to set PEL's for concentrations of chemicals in
workplace air.

Workers may receive large doses by inhalation. A worker
exposed to an airborne contaminant (molecular weight 170) at
a concentration of 10 ppm in workplace air will receive a
dose of about 10 mg/kg per work day, assuming an inhalation
volume of 10 cubic meters (10,000 liters) per 8-hour
workday, 70 kg body weight, and 100% absorption. The actual
absorption by the lung of inhaled solvents will be somewhat
less, varying between 40-70% (Astrand, 1976). PEL's for
many workplace carcinogens have ranged historically from 1-
1000 ppm. As a consequence, large doses of carcinogens
(0.1-100 mg/kg/day) may be received by inhalation (see Table
2).

Inhalation bioassays provide the best estimates of EPI
values for volatile carcinogens. Such bioassays are not
common. Recent results from well-designed lifetime
inhalation bioassays for 9 major industrial substances have
become available: five sponsored by the National Toxicology
Program (NTP), and one apiece sponsored by the American
Petroleum Institute (API), Chemical Industry Institute of
Technology (CIIT), National Institute of Industrial Health
of Japan, and Union Carbide (see Table 1).

We have calculated EPI values for these 9 substances using
the carcinogenic dose (CED) estimated from the inhalation
bioassays. Ideally, comparisons would be made among values
based on CED's for the same test animal and route of
administration, e.g. inhalation using male F344 rats. (It
is worth noting that the potency values for rats and mice
are highly correlated among chemicals which are carcinogenic
to both species (Bernstein, et al, 1984).) It would be
instructive to compare EPI values from inhalation studies
with those from ingestion studies.

DISCUSSION

EPI values have been calculated for 9 volatile industrial
compounds using both the old and the new regulatory
standards. Several conclusions can be drawn from
comparisons of the EPI values for these substances.

The EPI is Useful in Identifying Priority Chemicals for Regulatory Action

When these compounds are ranked according to the EPI values
for current Federal Permissible Exposure Limits, 1,3-
butadiene and formaldehyde are priority candidates for
regulatory action (see Table 2). This ranking is based on
figures which assume that workers have similar full-time
exposures to the various PEL's, and does not adjust for the
slope of the dose-response curve estimated from the animal
studies.

TABLE 1.   Inhalation Bioassays of 9 Major Industrial Chemicals Used to
           Calculate EPI's

Chemical	Bioassay (References)	Test Animal Sex/Str/Species	Target Site	Proportion of Animals with Tumors[a] (%)
1,3-Butadiene	NTP (13)	m B6C3F1 mice	malignant lymphoma	45
1,2-Dibromo-3-Chloropropane	NTP (14)	m F344 rat	nasal carcinoma	60
1,2-Dibromo-ethane	NTP (15)	m F344 rat	nasal adeno-carcinoma	40
Ethylene Oxide	Union(20) Carbide	f F344 rat	mononuclear-cell leukemia	50
Formaldehyde	CIIT (3)	m F344 rat	nasal carcinoma	50
Unleaded Gasoline	API (11)	m SD rat	mixed renal tumors	5
Methylene Chloride	NTP (16)	m B6C3F1 mice	lung carcinoma	50
Propylene Oxide	NTP (17)	m B6C3F1 mice	nasal hem/hes[b]	20
Trichloroethylene	NIIH (8)	f ICR mice	lung adeno-carcinoma	15

a   Animals with tumors = (incidence in dosed animals) - (incidence in
    control animals), for the specified target site.

b   Nasal cavity hemangioma and hemangiosarcoma.

<u>Workers Have Been Permitted to be Exposed to Doses Which are
Close to Those That Produce Cancer in Test Animals</u>

For four of the chemicals (1,2-dibromoethane (EDB), ethylene
oxide, 1,3-butadiene, and formaldehyde), workers were
legally permitted to be exposed at some time to dose levels
that were greater than 25% of the dose which induced tumors
in laboratory animals (see Table 2).

<u>Lowered PEL's Have Markedly Reduced the EPI Values for
Several Important Industrial Chemicals</u>

Changes in the PEL's for 1,2-dibromoethane (EDB) and
ethylene oxide (and additionally in California for methylene
chloride and trichloroethylene) have resulted in marked
reductions in EPI values. In the case of EDB, this
reduction was greater than 100-fold. As a result, full-time
workplace exposures to 1,3-butadiene and formaldehyde at the
current PEL present the potential for
greater danger than are similar exposures, for example, to
DBCP, EDB, and TCE (see Table 2).

<u>The Margin of Protection Provided by the PEL for Different
Chemicals Has Varied Over 1000-Fold</u>

EPI values for the 9 carcinogens are presented in Table 2.
These values have varied over 1000-fold during the past 5
years (in 1980, EDB = 231; DBCP = 0.2). Thus, there has
been considerable variation in the margin of protection
provided to workers for these chemicals.

<u>Some State Standards (PEL's) Are Considerably More
Protective Than Federal Standards (PEL's)</u>

Standards set by the State of California are considerably
more stringent in several cases than those at the Federal
level (e.g. PEL's for methylene chloride, propylene oxide,
and trichloroethylene are 4-5 fold lower in California: see
Table 3). However, even California's PEL's may not provide
adequate protection: for some chemicals, California workers
are still permitted to receive up to 36% of the dose that
produced cancer in test animals (see Table 2).

<u>Accurate Information Is Needed on the Numbers of Workers
Exposed to Specific Substances and the Levels of Their
Exposures</u>

Such information can be coupled with EPI values to identify
potential problems for populations of workers and to rank
them on a priority scale for corrective action. The best
estimates of the numbers of U.S. workers exposed either
full-time or part-time to specific chemicals are provided by

TABLE 2.   Inhalation EPI Values, for Nine Major Industrial Chemical
           Carcinogens, Ranked According to the EPI for the Current Federal
           PEL

Chemical		PEL[a] (mg/M3)	OED:[b] Occupational Effective Dose (mg/kg/day)	CED:[c] Cancer Effective Dose[d] (mg/kg/day)	EPI: OED CED X 100 ($)
1,3-Butadiene		2200	126	346	36
Formaldehyde	U.S.	3.7	.25	0.9	28
	Cal.	2.5	.15		17
Trichloro-	U.S.	540	30.8	[971]	[3.2]
ethylene	Cal.	135	7.7		[0.8]
Methylene	U.S.	1800	103	3702	2.8
Chloride	Cal.	360	20.6		0.6
Unleaded Gasoline		900	52	[2086]	[2.5]
Propylene	U.S.	240	14	[642]	[2.2]
Oxide	Cal.	50	2.9		[0.4]
1,2-Dibromoethane		1 (153)	0.06 (8.8)	3.8	1.5 (231)
Ethylene Oxide		1.8 (90)	0.1 (5.2)	13	0.8 (40)
1,2-Dibromo-3-chloropropane		0.01	0.0006	0.3	0.2

a PEL = Permissible Exposure Limit (mg/M3): permitted concentrations in
   workplace air, either (old) or current values. Values are for Federal
   PEL's, except where California is different and is noted separately. Old
   PEL's (mg/M3) which have been revised downward are in ( ).

b OED = Occupational Effective Dose: workplace dose by inhalation that
   workers may receive at the current PEL; calculated from Eqn. 2 using
   values for inhalation volume and body weight in humans of 10,000
   liters/8-hr day, 70 kg; assumes a 40-year worklife, 70-year lifespan, and
   100$ absorption. Values in ( ) are calculated from old PEL's which have
   been revised downward.

c CED = Cancer Effective Dose: chronic dose by inhalation that produced
   significant (p<0.05) increases in tumors in test animals; calculated from
   Eqn. 2 using values for inhalation volumes and body weights in rodents:
   male rats, 0.1 l/min, 0.5 kg; female rats, 0.1 l/min, 0.35 kg; male and
   female mice, 0.03 l/min, 0.03 kg; assumes 100$ absorption (Gold, et al.
   1984.

d Values in brackets [ ] have been adjusted to approximate the dose that
   induces tumors in 50$ of the animals.

Table 3.   Permissible Exposure Limits in ppm, EPI Values, and the Estimated
           Number of Workers Exposed to Each of 9 Industrial Chemicals

Chemical	PEL in ppm U.S.	PEL in ppm Calif	EPI Based on on Current PEL[a] U.S.	EPI Based on on Current PEL[a] Calif	Number of U.S. Workers[b] Part-time	Number of U.S. Workers[b] Full-time
1,3-Butadiene	1000		36		45,000	15,000
Formaldehyde	3	2	28	17	488,000	28,000
Trichloroethylene	100	25	[3.2]	[0.8]	507,000	11,000
Methylene Chloride	500	100	2.8	0.6	843,000	7,000
Unleaded Gasoline	300		[2.5]		1,095,000	19,000
Propylene Oxide	100	20	[2.2]	[0.4]	39,000	400
1,2-Dibromoethane	0.13		1.5		6,300	none
Ethylene Oxide	1		0.8		96,000	none
1,2-Dibromo-3-Chloropropane	0.001		0.2		350	none

a [ ] Values are adjusted to the approximate dose that induces tumors in 50%
  of the animals.

b Data derived from National Occupational Hazard Survey (NOHS) of 1972-74.
  National Institute of Occupational Safety and Health, Pers. Comm. D.
  Sundin, 1985.   Part-time is a minimum cumulative exposure of more than 30
  minutes per week for 90% of the work weeks per year; and up to 4 hours per
  day. Full-time is more than 4 hour per day. Figures subject to sizable
  standard errors, especially for small numbers. Figures for some chemicals
  (e.g., trichloroethylene) may now be much lower due to market
  substitution. Gasoline includes leaded and unleaded.

the National Occupational Hazard Survey (NOHS) (NIOSH,
1977). Chemicals with extensive worker exposure (e.g.
methylene chloride) may be priority candidates for
corrective action even though they do not have the highest
EPI values (see Table 3).

ACKNOWLEDGEMENTS

The authors gratefully acknowledge discussions with Richard
Peto and the assistance of Renae Magaw, Will Hevelin, and
Yolanda Apodaca.

REFERENCES

1. Ames, B.N., Hooper, K., Sawyer, C.B., Friedman, A.D.,
    Peto, R., Havender, W., Gold, L.S., Haggin, T., Harris,
    R.H., and Rosenfeld, M.: Carcinogenic Potency: A
    Progress Report. In: Banbury Report 5. Ethylene
    Dichloride: A Potential Health Risk?, edited by B. Ames,
    P. Infante, and R. Reitz, pp. 55-63. Cold Spring Harbor
    Laboratory, Cold Spring Harbor, NY, 1980.

2. Astrand, I. and Ovrum, P.: Exposure to trichloroethylene
    I: Uptake and Distribution in man. Scand. J. Work
    Environ. Health 4:199-211, 1976.

3. Battelle, Columbus Laboratories: A Chronic Inhalation
    Toxicity Study in Rats and Mice Exposed to Formaldehyde.
    Battelle, Columbus Laboratories, Columbus, OH, 1981.

4. Bernstein, L., Gold, L.S., Ames, B.N., Pike, M.C. and
    Hoel, D.G. Some tautologous aspects of carcinogenic
    potency in rats and mice. Fundamental and Appl.
    Toxicol. 5:70-86, 1985.

5. California Occupational Safety and Health Administration
    (Cal/OSHA): Airborne Contaminants, General Industry
    Safety Order #5155, Title 8, California Administrative
    Code, Cal/OSHA, Department of Industrial Relations, San
    Francisco, 1984.

6. California Occupational Safety and Health Administration
    (Cal/OSHA): Occupational Carcinogens, General Industry
    Safety Orders #5208-5215 and 5217-5219, Title 8,
    California Administrative Code, Cal/OSHA, Department of
    Industrial Relations, San Francisco, 1984.

7. Crouch, E. and Wilson, R.: Interspecies Comparison of
    Carcinogenic Potency. J.Toxicol. Environ. Health
    5:1095-1118, 1979.

8. Fukuda, K. Takemoto, K., and Tsuruta, H.: Inhalation
    Carcinogenicity of Trichloroethylene in Mice and Rats.
    Indust. Hlth. 21:243-254, 1983.

9. Gold, L.S., Sawyer, C. B., Magaw, R., Backman, G.M., de
    Veciana, M., Levinson, R., Hooper, N.K., Havender, W.R.,
    Bernstein, L., Peto, R., Pike, M.C., and Ames, B.N.: A
    carcinogenic potency data-base of the standardized
    results of animal bioassays. Environ. Health Persp.
    58:9-319, 1984.

10. International Agency for Research on Cancer (IARC): IARC
    Monographs on the Evaluation of the Carcinogenic Risk of
    Chemicals to Humans, Vols. 1-38, IARC, World Health
    Organization, Lyon, France, 1971-1985.

11. MacFarland, H.N.: Xenobiotic Induced Kidney Lesions:
    Hydrocarbons. The 90-Day and 2-Year Gasoline Studies.
    In: Advances in Modern Environmental Toxicology, Vol.
    VII, Renal Effects of Petroleum Hydrocarbons, edited by
    M.A. Mehlman, C.P. Hemstreet, III, J.J. Thorpe, and N.K.
    Weaver, pp. 51-56. Princeton, Princeton Scientific
    Publishers, 1984.

12. Meselson, M. and Russell, K.: Comparisons of
    Carcinogenic and Mutagenic Potency. In: Origins of
    Human Cancer, edited by H. Hiatt, J.D. Watson, and J.A.
    Winsten, pp. 1473-1482. Cold Spring Harbor Conference
    on Cell Proliferation. Cold Spring Harbor Laboratory,
    Cold Spring Harbor, NY, 1977.

13. National Toxicology Program Technical Report Series, No.
    288: Toxicology and Carcinogenesis Studies of 1,3-
    Butadiene in B6C3F1 Mice (Inhalation Studies). NIH
    Publication No. 84-2544, National Toxicology Program,
    National Institutes of Health, Public Health Service,
    U.S. Department of Health and Human Services, 1984.

14. National Toxicology Program Technical Report Series, No.
    206: Carcinogenesis Bioassay of 1,2-Dibromo-3-
    Chloropropane in F344 Rats and B6C3F1 Mice (Inhalation
    Study). NIH Publication No. 82-1762, National
    Toxicology Program, National Institutes of Health,
    Public Health Service, U.S. Department of Health and
    Human Services, 1982.

15. National Toxicology Program Technical Report Series, No.
    210: Bioassay of 1,2-Dibromoethane for Possible
    Carcinogenicity. NIH Publication No. 82-1766,
    Carcinogenesis Testing Program, National Cancer
    Institute, and National Toxicology Program, National
    Institutes of Health, Public Health Service, U.S.
    Department of Health and Human Services, 1982.

16. National Toxicology Program Technical Report, Approved
    Final Draft: Toxicology and Carcinogenesis Studies of
    Dichloromethane (Methylene Dichloride) in F344/N Rats
    and B6C3F1 Mice (Inhalation Studies). National
    Toxicology Program, National Institutes of Health,
    Public Health Service, U.S. Department of Health and
    Human Services, 1985.

17. National Toxicology Program Technical Report Series, No.
    267: Toxicology and Carcinogenesis Studies of Propylene
    Oxide in F344 Rats and B6C3F1 Mice (Inhalation Studies).
    NIH Publication No. 85-2527, National Toxicology
    Program, National Institutes of Health, Public Health
    Service, U.S. Department of Health and Human Services,
    1985.

18. Office of Science and Technology Policy (OSTP):
    Chemical Carcinogens; A Review of the Science and Its
    Associated Principles. Office of Science and Technology
    Policy, Executive Office of the President, 1985.

19. Peto, R., Pike, M.C., Bernstein, L., Gold, L.S., and
    Ames, B.N. The TD50: A proposed general convention for
    the numerical description of the carcinogenic potency of
    chemicals in chronic-exposure animal experiments.
    Environ. Health Perspect. 58:1-8, 1984.

20. Snellings, W.M., Pringle, J.L., Dorko, J.D., and
    Kintigh, W.J.: Teratology and Reproduction Studies with
    Rats Exposed to 10, 33, or 100 ppm of Ethylene Oxide
    (ETO). J. Ind. Hyg. and Tox. 31:A84 (Abstract), 1979.

3

Can Cancer Be Prevented?

ED CADMAN

INTRODUCTION

Cancer will be diagnosed in nearly 1.2 million people this year in the United States. Nearly half of these individuals will be cured of their cancer by surgical resection of the tumor before metastasis has occurred. Of the nearly 600,000 patients who will have disseminated cancer, close to 50,000 patients will be cured by chemotherapy, often in combination with radiation therapy. It is apparent from these figures that treatment of cancer is only helpful to perhaps 50% of all patients with this disease. The other approach is to prevent the cancer from developing. However, for the best success at prevention, we must understand the mechanism by which the cancer is caused. By understanding the cause, preventive measures can be made rather specific.

It is well understood that many agents can induce a malignant change of a cell in the laboratory. These carcinogens are considered to cause this malignant transformation by altering the structure of the DNA and therefore changing the message contained by the proper DNA sequence of bases. These concepts are represented in Figures 1 and 2.

MESSAGE OF DNA CONTROLS CELL

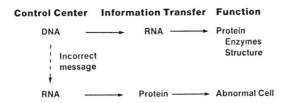

FIGURE 1. The DNA contains the code which, when translated by RNA into proteins, results in cellular structure and function. Any alteration in this code or transfer process can lead to incorrect proteins and result in an abnormal cell.

HOW DO CHEMICALS AFFECT DNA?

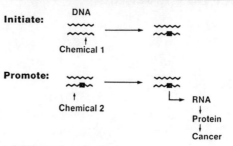

- Intitiator causes damage
- Promoter results in the message transfer

FIGURE 2. Chemicals can affect the DNA in two major ways. Certain chemicals may lead to a DNA change which is not translated by RNA into an abnormal protein. These chemicals are referred to as initiators. Other chemicals may promote the subsequent translation process of this altered DNA segment resulting in the abnormal protein and the development of the abnormal cell. These agents are considered promoters.

Therefore, to prevent cancer from developing, compounds could be segregated into two main classes -- those which prevent the DNA damage, or those which counteract the abnormal product made as a consequence of the altered DNA. These agents, referred to as initiators, cause an initial lesion in the DNA and by themselves may not result in cancer until a second agent alters the DNA in some unknown fashion, thus promoting the malignant transformation process (Fig. 3). In both instances, preventive

MECHANISM OF PREVENTING CANCER

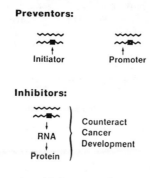

FIGURE 3. Agents which prevent cancer could influence at least three areas of chemical carcinogenesis. They could interfere with the initiator process, for example, by detoxifying the carcinogen prior to interaction with the DNA, or by interfering with the binding of the carcinogen to the DNA. Initiator actions of a preventing agent would also affect promoting carcinogenesis. In addition, certain agents could inhibit the transfer process (RNA) or the abnormal protein, thus preventing the expression of the abnormal coded DNA from affecting the cell.

substances would be useful. For example, if a known agent were an initiator and this agent were prevalent in a particular occupation, and if we also knew that a cancer would only develop following the subsequent exposure of a promoting agent, then perhaps a compound could be given which would prevent the action of the promoter. The result would of course be the prevention of cancer. If there were preventive compounds which interfered with the action of the initiating carcinogen, then the adminstering of such compounds could also prevent cancer.

These concepts are extremely important, since it has been estimated that between 70% and 90% of all cancers are due to agents within our environment and diet. If this is true, then prevention is the most reasonable approach for avoiding cancer. This implies therefore that if the causative agents are so prevalent, the preventive agents would then need to be given to the entire population so as to effectively reduce the incidence of cancer. Preventive agents must therefore be taken on a regular basis, as well as be virtually non-toxic. There are a few substances which may be useful in the prevention of cancer.

VITAMIN A

Vitamin A is available as a retinol or as a beta-carotene. Vitamin A can reduce the prevalence of tumors in certain experimental animals (1). However, the more important cancer preventive agent has been considered the carotenes. There have been many population studies reported which have demonstrated an association between high vitamin A levels or intake and reduced cancer (2-7). The major influence appears to be with lung cancer and squamous cell malignancies.

There have been two recent prospective evaluations comparing stored serum samples for retinol concentrations with cancer. It was of interest that there was an increased incidence of lung cancer in these individuals with low retinol levels (8,9). Other similar studies have not found such an association (10,11). A recent review of five prospective and fifteen retrospective studies by Peto et al. have noted a consistent association between a lower cancer incidence and higher than average beta-carotene levels (12). A more recent study has also found a similar beneficial effect of beta-carotene ingestion and reduced lung cancer (13).

An important experimental observation is that the protective effect of these retinols can be observed even when they are given well after the administration of a carcinogen (14). This is important because it implies that the retinols could prevent the induction of malignancy at a time substantially after the exposure to a cancer-causing agent.

Vitamin C and Vitamin E

Both of these vitamins can act as antioxidants. Free radicals and singlet oxygen are quite toxic to many biological chemicals and structures. For example, many carcinogens alter the structure of the DNA molecule by the intermediate formation of these toxic substances. Therefore, any agent which would reduce free radicals and singlet oxygen could potentially reduce the incidence of cancer which is the result of altered DNA structures. Although there are insufficient data available on humans to evaluate this hypothesis, vitamin E does appear capable of reducing the incidence of tumors in animals (15,16).

In addition to the antioxidant effects of vitamin C, other actions have been cited as potential reasons why this vitamin might prevent cancer (17). Nitroso compounds have been definitely associated with cancer. Vitamin C does prevent the production of these carcinogens from nitrates, which are common in our diet (18,19). Experimental animal studies have confirmed this anti-cancer effect of vitamin C. However, there is no useful available information correlating vitamin C and human cancers, although such studies are in progress.

SELENIUM

This metal has been associated with cancer in that low levels or low direct intake have been associated with higher than expected cancer rates. Many animal studies have demonstrated a protective effect of selenium on cancer development from several different carcinogens (21). Selenium is required for the action of the enzyme glutathione peroxidase. This enzyme is important for the reduction of toxic H_2O_2 to non-toxic H_2O and O_2. Therefore, this metal may be acting in a similar fashion biochemically as vitamins E and C.

INDOLES

Indoles are compounds which can induce the enzyme arylhydrocarbon hydroxylase which can metabolize the polycyclic hydrocarbons. The polycyclic hydrocarbons are well known carcinogens and have been implicated in the etiology of lung and colon cancers. The foods which contain high quantities of indoles are cabbage, brussel sprouts, broccoli and cauliflower and, in fact, an epidemiologic study has suggested that individuals who eat these vegetables have a reduced incidence of colon cancer (22). This has led to the recent suggestion by the American Cancer Society that these foods be consumed on a regular basis.

DIET

Dietary fat and fiber content and colon cancer have generated a great deal of concern during the last decade. Generally, the available studies have demonstrated that high fat and low fiber diets are associated with higher colon cancer rates than those diets which contain low fat and high fiber content (23). It must be appreciated that this is only a trend. There are numerous examples where this association was not found. Based on this information, one can conclude that dietary fat and fiber are probably important contributors to our health, but are not exclusive preventers or causes of colon cancer. High-fat diets have also been associated with other cancers as well. For example, obese women have a higher incidence of breast cancer.

It is well known that cigarettes and alcohol are associated with cancer development. The cancers which have been found to be increased in individuals who use these substances (24) in excess are lung, esophagus, kidney, and head and neck.

SUMMARY

There is little doubt that carcinogens are in our environment, and that our biologic system has sophisticated ways of detoxifying many of these compounds. To improve our health and reduce our chances for developing cancer, certain guidelines are useful. Eat in moderation a balanced diet which is low in fat, high in fiber, and which has adequate vitamin C, E, selenium-and indole-containing foods. Perhaps the most important advice is to avoid cigarettes and the excessive use of alcohol. The use of chemopreventive agents for cancer is a major field of interest for many investigators and is considered by the National Cancer Institute as a very worthy area for research (25).

REFERENCES

1. Saffiotti U, Montesano R, Sellakumar AR, Borg SA: Experimental cancer of the lung. Inhibition by vitamin A of the induction of tracheo-bronchial squamous metaplasia and squamous cell tumors. Cancer 20: 857-864, 1967.

2. Bjelke E: Dietary vitamin A and human lung cancer. Int J Cancer 15: 561-565, 1975.

3. Mettlin C, Grahm S, Swanson M: Vitamin A and lung cancer. J Natl Cancer Inst 62: 1435-1438, 1979.

4. Hirayam T: Diet and cancer. Nutr Cancer 1: 67-81, 1979.

5. MacLennan R, DaCosta NE, Law CH, Ng YK: Risk factors for lung cancer in Singapore Chinese. A population with high female incidence rates. Int J Cancer 20: 854-860, 1977.

6. Mettlin C, Graham S: Dietary risk factors in human bladder cancer. Am J Epidemiol 110: 255-263, 1979.

7. Shekelle RB, Lepper M, Liu S, Maliza C, Raynor WJ Jr, Rossof AH, Paul O, MacMilan Shyrock A, Stamler J: Dietary vitamin A and risk of cancer in the Western Electric study. Lancet ii: 1185-1190, 1981.

8. Wald N, Idle M, Boreham J, Bailey A: Low serum-vitamin A and subsequent risk of cancer: Preliminary results of a prospective study. Lancet ii: 813-815, 1980.

9. Kark JD, Smith AH, Switzer BR, Hames CG: Serum vitamin A (retinol) and cancer incidence in Evans County, Georgia. J Natl Cancer Inst 66: 7-16, 1981.

10. Willett WC, Polk F, Underwood BA, Stampfer MJ, Pressel S, Rosner B, Taylor JO, Schneider K, Hames CG: Relation of serum vitamin A and E and carotenoids to the risk of cancer. N Engl J Med 310: 430-434, 1984.

11. Wald NJ, Boreham J, Haywood JL, Bulbrook RD: Plasma retinol, beta-carotene and vitamin E levels in relation to the future risk of breast cancer. Br J Cancer 49: 321-3224, 1984.

12. Peto R, Doll R, Buckley JD, Spron MB: Can dietary beta-carotene materially reduce human cancer rates? Natur 290: 201-208, 1981.

13. Shekelle RB, Lepper M, Liu S, Maliza C, Raynor WJ Jr, Rossof AH: Dietary vitamin A and risk of cancer in the Western Electric study. Lancet ii: 1185-1190, 1981.

14. McCormick DL, Burns FJ, Albert RE: Inhibition of Benzo(a)pyrene induced mammary carcinogenesis by retinyl acetate. J Natl Cancer Inst 66: 559-564, 1981.

15. Cook MG, McNamara P: Effect of dietary vitamin E on dimethylhydrazine-induced colonic tumors in mice. Cancer Res 40: 1329, 1980.

16. Haber SL, Wissler RW: Effect of vitamin E on carcinogenicity of methylcholanthrene. Proc Soc Exp Biol Med 111: 774-775, 1962.

17. Cameron E, Wissler RW: Ascorbic acid and cancer: A review. Cancer Res 39: 663-681, 1979.

18. Mirvish SS, Wallcave L, Eagan M, Shubik P: Ascorbate-nitrate reaction: possible means of blocking the formation of carcinogenic N-nitroso compounds. Science 177: 65-68, 1972.

19. Mirvish SS, Cardesa A, Wallcave L, Shubik P: Induction of mouse lung adenomas by amines or ureas plus nitrite and by N-nitroso compounds: Effect of ascorbate, gallic acid, thiocyanate, and caffeine. J Natl Cancer Inst 55: 633-636, 1975.

20. Wattenberg LW: Inhibition of carcinogenic and toxic effects of polycyclic hydrocarbons by phenolic antioxidants and ethoxquin. J Natl Cancer Inst 48: 425-430, 1982.

21. Helzlsouer KJ: Selenium and cancer prevention. Semin Oncol 10(3): 305, 1983.

22. Graham S, Dayal H, Swanson M, Mittelman A, Wilkinson G: Diet in the epidemiology of cancer of the colon and rectum. J Natl Cancer Inst 61: 709-714, 1978.

23. Wynder EL, Reddy BS: Dietary fat and fiber and colon cancer. Semin Oncol 10(3): 264, 1983.

24. Broitman SA, Vitale JJ, Gottlieb LS: Ethanolic beverage consumption, cigarette smoking, nutritional status, and digestive tract cancers. Semin Oncol 10(3): 322, 1983.

25. Wattenberg LW: Chemoprevention of Cancer. Cancer Res 45: 1-8, 1985.

4

Pesticides, Viruses, and Sunlight in the Etiology of Cancer among Agricultural Workers

MARC SCHENKER and STEPHEN McCURDY

INTRODUCTION

It is commonly believed that the outdoor agricultural workplace is a healthful one. However, agricultural workers are exposed to numerous chemical, physical and biologic factors in performing their occupational activities. Three of these categories of agents-- pesticides, viruses, and sunlight--have been the focus of numerous studies as possible cancer-causing agents.[1]

Pesticides are a major source of public concern because of their pervasiveness in the environment, and because they are viewed as a possible cause of cancer.[2] Pesticide use is the most intensive in the agricultural setting, and studies of agricultural workers are a valuable tool to assess their potential association with cancer. Other potentially hazardous chemical agents to which farmers are exposed include herbicides, solvents, oils, detergents, and creosote.

Viruses are another exogenous agent being studied intensively in the laboratory as a cause of cancer. The agricultural workplace again provides a useful setting for epidemiologic studies of cancer and exposure to viral agents, particularly viral agents associated with farm animals. Finally, agriculture represents one of several occupations with increased exposure to sunlight, and is mentioned here because of it's contribution to increased skin cancer rates among farmers. The chapter by Mathias in this volume gives more detailed consideration of epidemiologic and experimental evidence concerning sunlight and skin cancer, and this subject will only briefly be considered further in the present chapter.

Epidemiologic studies have consistently observed a lower overall standardised mortality rate among farmers. Selection of healthier people to work in agriculture and lifestyle factors may explain this finding.[3] Farming is a physically demanding occupation; less healthy, unfit persons are not likely to become farmers. Those who become ill as farmers may switch to less difficult lines of work,

leaving the more fit individuals to pursue farming. An important
lifestyle factor is the lower prevalence of smoking among farmers.[4]
Mortality studies have found decreased rates of certain tobacco-
associated tumors among farmers. Burmeister[5] observed significantly
decreased proportionate mortality from cancers of the lung
(PMR=0.78), esophagus (PMR=0.74), and buccal cancers other than lip
(PMR=0.82). Significant decreases in PMR's for cancers of the lung
were also seen among farmers in the mortality surveys undertaken in
California and Washington.[6,7]

Despite lower overall and smoking-related mortality rates, studies
of farmers have found increased mortality rates for some specific
malignancies. In a study of 6402 Iowa farmers dying between 1971
and 1978, Burmeister[5] found statistically significant elevations of
the proportionate mortality ratios (PMR) from cancer of the lip
(PMR=1.62), leukemia (PMR=1.10), lymphoma (PMR=1.14), multiple
myeloma (PRM=1.27), prostatic carcinoma (PMR=1.10), and stomach
cancer (PMR=1.14). Increased PMR's for non-melanoma skin cancers
have been found among farmers from California (PMR=1.55, p<0.05) and
Washington (PMR=1.36, p<0.05).[6]

While large mortality surveys must be considered hypothesis generat-
ing, and significant associations may occur by chance alone, the
consistency of increased mortality rates for certain cancers among
farmers is noteworthy. The remainder of this chapter will discuss
some of the epidemiologic data pertaining to specific cancers among
agriculture workers or associated with known agriculture exposures
such as pesticides.

Leukemia

An increased risk or mortality ratio for leukemia has frequently
been observed among farmers. Burmeister[5] found a PMR of 1.10
(p<0.05) for leukemia among Iowa farmers. The large occupational
mortality study in Washington state noted a PMR of 1.08 among general farmers, which was not statistically significant.[7] Among wheat
farmers and poultry farmers the PMR's for leukemia were 1.47 and
2.69, respectively (p<0.05).

A weakness of the PMR is that the sum of the proportionate mortalities must equal one. Thus, a decreased risk for mortality from one
cause may be accompanied by a spurious increase in mortality from
other causes. This is of concern in studies of farmers because they
have a lower risk for smoking-related causes of death. Some of the
increased PMR from non-smoking-related diseases (such as leukemia)
may be due to decreases in smoking-related disorders such as lung
cancer.

Case-control studies of leukemia have also found an association of
farming and leukemia. Blair[8] found an odds ratio of 1.25 (p<0.05)
for farming among 1084 leukemia deaths and matched controls occurring in Nebraska between 1957 and 1974. Similar results were
obtained by Milham[9] in Washington and Oregon, and by Blair[10] in
Wisconsin. A case-control study in Minnesota[11] failed to detect an
increased odds ratio for farming among leukemia cases, but

this was a small study and may not have had adequate power to observe an association if it were present.

A pattern of increased risk of leukemia in younger cases and an association with certain farming practices suggests that recently introduced farming methods may play a role in the increased leukemia rates of farmers.[12] One such change is the introduction of large amounts of synthetic pesticides and herbicides to farming over the past four decades. Since many of these compounds are known to be carcinogenic under laboratory conditions, attention has been focused on these chemicals as a possible causal factor. However, the epidemiologic data do not yet establish a causal role for these substances.

Increased exposure to leukemogenic viruses has also been hypothesised to be a cause of leukemia among farmers. Viruses are known to cause lymphoreticular malignancies in several animal models including cows (bovine lymphosarcoma virus) and chickens (fowl leukosis virus).[13] A viral etiology has been shown for cerain T-cell leukemias in humans.[14] Although carcinogenic animal viruses have not been demonstrated to cause human cancer, some epidemiological evidence invites speculation.

Blair[16] found an odds ratio of 1.18 (not significant, p>0.05) for farming among leukemia cases from Wisconsin counties with high chicken populations. An odds ratio of 1.53 (p<0.05) was observed for farming among leukemia cases born after 1900 in the 33 Iowa counties with the highest inventories of egg-laying chickens, but the association did not hold for cases born between 1890 and 1900.[15] Milham reported an increased risk of leukemia among poultry farmers in Washington state.[9] This association was not noted among Nebraska farmers.[8]

Modes of infection for leukemogenic viruses may include direct contact with infected animals, through a common vector, or through contaminated milk products. A role for this agent is supported by the results of a study in Iowa[16] showing a correlation between rates for acute lymphatic leukemia(ALL) and dairying activity. The ALL rates were highest in those counties with herds known to be infected with the bovine lymphosarcoma virus. However, a seroepidemiological investigation did not find antibody to this virus among farmers, veterinarians, or leukemia patients.[17]

Polish investigators have reported an association between leukemia rates in cattle and human hospital admission rates for leukemia.[18] However, no such association was detected in similar studies from Sweden[19], or the U.S.S.R.[1] A role for a leukemogenic virus would be further supported by a finding that the increase in leukemia among farmers was restricted to a single histological type. Unfortunately a clear and consistent association has not been shown. Statistically significant associations have been found between farming and chronic lymphatic[15], unspecified lymphatic[15], and unspecified acute leukemias[8]. Investigation is made somewhat difficult by inadequacies in the 7th ICD classification codes for leukemias. For example, both acute lymphatic and acute myeloid leukemias may appear under the same code (204.3).[20]

In summary, several lines of evidence have suggested an association
between farming and leukemia. Although leukemogenic viruses and
newer farming practices such as synthetic chemical use may be con-
tributory, the epidemiologic evidence is not consistent and does not
prove a causal role.

Soft Tissue Sarcoma

Isolated case reports relating phenoxyacetic acids, chlorophenols,
and contaminants to soft tissue sarcomas have led to an increased
interest in the carcinogenic potentials of these compounds in the
agricultural setting.[21]   Phenoxyacetic acids are a class of herbicides including 2,4-dichlorophenoxyacetic acid (2,4-D), 4-chloro-2-
methyl phenoxyacetic acid (MCPA), and 2,4,5-trichlorophenoxyacetic
acid (2,4,5-T). In Sweden the phenoxyacetic acids are commonly used
as herbicides in forestry applications to control unwanted hard-
woods. MCPA is a commonly used herbicide in agriculture. These
agents were also used in Viet Nam as constituents of "Agent Orange".
Chlorophenols have been used as fungicides in the production of
paper pulp, and as an impregnate to prevent staining in freshly sawn
wood.

Hardell and Sandstrom[22] performed a case-control study in Sweden to
test the association between soft tissue sarcomas and these compounds. They studied 21 living and 31 deceased cases, and controls
selected from the general population matched 4:1 on sex, age, and
municipality of residence. Living cases were matched with living
controls and deceased cases with controls dying within one year of
the death of the respective case. Those dying of cancer were
excluded from the control population for deceased cases. An odds
ratio of 5.7 (p<0.001) was observed among cases for exposure to
these compounds.

The association observed in this study may in part be due to carcinogenic effects of substances which are often found as impurities in
preparations of chlorophenols and phenoxyacetic acids, such as
polychlorinated dibenzodioxins and dibenzofurans. These are often
found in chlorophenols and 2,4,5-T, whereas other phenoxyacetic
acids such as 2,4-D and MCPA are generally free of these contaminants. A Swedish follow-up study[23] involving 110 incident cases of
soft tissue sarcoma and 219 controls in southern Sweden showed a
comparably increased odds ratio (OR=6.8, p<0.05) for exposure to
phenoxyacetic acids, including non-2,4,5-T phenoxyacetic acids considered free from impurities.

A case-control study from the New Zealand Cancer Registry[24] failed
to confirm the association of exposure to phenoxyacetic acids and
soft tissue sarcoma. This study of 82 cases and 92 controls differed from the Swedish investigations in that the control population
consisted solely of patients with other tumors. An odds ratio of
1.3 for exposure was noted among cases, which was not statistically
significant. Possible explanations for the differing results
between the Swedish and New Zealand investigations include impuri-

ties or co-carcinogenic factors present in the Swedish environment
or chemical preparations that are absent in New Zealand. The methodological differences may also be important. If phenoxyacetic acids
and chlorophenols cause other types of malignancies besides soft
tissue sarcomas, then the utilisation of patients with other tumors
for controls (as in the New Zealand study) would dilute a true positive correlation. Selective recall for herbicide exposure may have
occurred in the Scandinavian sarcoma cases, contributing to the
elevated odds ratio for association.

In summary, an association between soft tissue sarcoma and exposure
to phenoxyacetic acids, chlorophenols and contaminant compounds is
supported by case-control investigations in Sweden, but a New Zealand study did not confirm these results. Concern about a causal
association is supported by soft-tissue sarcoma cases among workers
who manufacture phenoxyherbicides and related compounds.[21] Efforts
at minimising occupational exposure to these substances are clearly
appropriate, but further study is required to clarify their carcinogenic effects in the workplace.

Lymphoma and Multiple Myeloma

Several investigators have noted an association between farming and
lymphomas (both Hodgkins's and non-Hodgkin's) and multiple myeloma.
Peterson and Milham[6] found a PMR of 1.34 for Hodgkin's lymphoma
among California farm workers dying between 1959 and 1961. In a
case-control study of 774 patients and controls in Wisconsin dying
of non-Hodgkin's lymphoma[25], an odds ratio of 1.22 for farming was
observed, which did not achieve statistical significance. Significant odds ratio elevations were noted, however, in patients dying
before age 65. The younger decedents were found to be at increased
risk for the reticulum cell sarcoma type of non-Hodgkin's lymphoma.
An association between farming and lymphoma and multiple myeloma has
also been noted in PMR and case-control studies in Iowa.[5,26]

Not all studies have found increased rates for lymphoma and multiple
myeloma among farm workers. A study of California patients dying of
lymphoma or multiple myeloma observed no significant increase of
standardised mortality ratios for these tumors among farmers.[27] This
investigation involved 3477 non-Hodgkin's lymphoma patients, 777
with Hodgkin's lymphoma, and 789 with multiple myeloma. A case-
control study in Washington and Oregon[8] also found no association
between farming and lymphomas. This study did detect a significant
association between farming and leukemia and between farming and
multiple myeloma.

Several investigators have attempted to discern specific risk factors associated with lymphoma or multiple myeloma among farmers.
Exposure to certain chemicals may be involved in the causation of
lymphomas and multiple myeloma. Cantor[25] noted increased risk for
non-Hodgkin's lymphoma in Wisconsin counties with increased small
grain acreage and insecticide use. Burmeister[26] found associations
between non-Hodgkin's lymphoma and counties with high inventories of
egg-laying chickens, milk products sold, hog production, and herbicide use. Multiple myeloma was associated with egg-laying chickens,

hog production, and insecticide and herbicide use.

Some specific chemical exposures have been implicated in lymphoma causation. A Swedish case-control study[28] of malignant lymphoma patients (Hodgkin's and non-Hodgkin's lymphoma) detected an elevated odds ratio of 6.0 ($p < 0.05$) for exposure to phenoxyacetic acids, or chlorophenols. Case reports in the U.S.A.[29] have implicated the nematocide 1,3 dichloropropene as a causal agent of lymphoma in acute overdoses, raising concern about exposures to this agent in the agricultural setting.

Prostatic Carcinoma

Several studies have found an increased risk of prostatic carcinoma among farmers. Williams and coworkers[30] utilised an interviewed sample of patients from the Third National Cancer Survey. An odds ratio of 1.52 ($p < 0.05$) for farming was observed among 379 cases of prostatic carcinoma and the control group of 1849 male patients with other tumors. A standardised mortality ratio of 1.95 ($p < 0.05$) for prostatic carcinoma was observed among white male farmers in Winnebago county, Illinois.[31] Burmeister[5] studied proportionate mortalities among Iowa farmers and found an increased PMR of 1.10 ($p < 0.05$) for prostatic cancer.

Evidence for specific high risk farming practices is contradictory. An association between poultry-raising activity and prostate cancer has been observed in Washington.[7] Blair[32] found a weak but statistically significant association with the number of chickens inventoried in a study of mortality rates for prostatic carcinoma in 3056 U.S. counties. A large death certificate study in Iowa[26] including 4827 cases of prostatic carcinoma and controls matched 2:1 on county of residence, age and calendar year of death observed an odds ratio of 1.19 ($p < 0.05$) for farming among cases. No correlation with poultry raising or other specific farming practices was detected.

In summary, several studies point to an association between farming and prostate cancer. The strength of this association, and possible influence of farming practices such as poultry raising does not appear to be great.

CONCLUSION

Epidemiological investigations have observed an association between farming and certain tumors including leukemia, lymphoma, multiple myeloma, and prostatic carcinoma. Although causal agents have yet to be confirmed, suspicion has been focused on occupational exposures to pesticides, herbicides, and zoonotic viruses. Study results are not consistent enough to support a causal role for these agents, but do emphasize the need for further research and to reduce occupational exposures when possible.

REFERENCES

1. Blair A: Cancer risks associated with agriculture: Epidemio-
    logical evidence. In: Genetic Toxicology, An Agricultural Per-
    spective, edited by RA Fleck, A Hollo, Basic Life Sciences vol
    21, p 93. New York, London, Plenum Press, 1982.

2. Sternberg SS: The carcinogenesis, mutagenesis, and terato-
    genesis of insecticides. Review of studies in animals and man.
    Pharmacol Ther 6:147-166, 1979.

3. Cassel J, Heyden S, Bartel AG, Kaplan BH, Tyroler HA, Cornoni
    JC, Hames CG: Occupation and physical activity and coronary
    heart disease. Arch Intern Med 128:920-928, 1971.

4. Sterling TD, Weinkam JJ: Smoking characteristics by type of
    employment. JOM 18:743-754, 1976.

5. Burmeister LF: Cancer mortality in Iowa farmers, 1971-78. JNCI
    66:461-464, 1981.

6. Peterson GR, Milham S: Occupational mortality in the state of
    California 1959-1961. DHEW Pub. no. (NIOSH, NIH) 80-104, Rock-
    ville, Maryland, 1980.

7. Milham S: Occupational mortality in Washington state, 1950-
    1971. DHEW Pub. no. (NIOSH, NIH) 76-175 A, Rockville, Mary-
    land, 1980.

8. Blair A, Thomas TL: Leukemia among Nebraska farmers: A death
    certificate study. Am J Epidemiol 110:264-273, 1979.

9. Milham S: Leukemia and multiple myeloma in farmers. Am J Epi-
    demiol 94:307-310, 1971.

10. Blair A, White DW: Death certificate study of leukemia among
    farmers from Wisconsin. JNCI 66:1027-1030, 1981.

11. Linos A, Kyle RA, O'Fallon WM, Kurland LT: A case-control study
    of occupational exposures and leukaemia. Int J Epedimiol
    9:131-135, 1980.

12. Archer VE: Cancer mortality in Iowa farmers. JNCI 67:743, 1981.

13. Heath CW, GG Caldwell, PC Feorino. Viruses and other microbes,
    In: Persons at high risk of cancer, edited by JF Fraumeni,
    Academic Press, New York, 1975

14. Broder S, Gallo RC: A pathogenic retrovirus (HTLV-III) linked
    to AIDS. N Engl J Med 311:1292-1297, 1984.

15. Burmeister LF, Van Lier SF, Isacson P: Leukemia and farm prac-
    tices in Iowa. Am J Epidemiol 115:720-728, 1982.

16. Donham KJ, Berg JW, Sawin RS: Epidemiologic relationships of the bovine populations and human leukemia in Iowa. Am J Epidemiol 112:80-92, 1980.

17. Donham KJ, VanDerMaaten MJ, Miller JM, Kruse BC, Rubino MJ: Seroepidemiologic studies on the possible relationships of human and bovine leukemia: brief communication. JNCI 59:851-853, 1977.

18. Wolska A: Human and bovine leukaemias. Lancet 1:1155, 1968.

19. Kvarnfors E, Henricson B, Hugoson G: A statistical study on farm and village level on the possible relations between human leukaemia and bovine leukosis. Acta Vet Scand 16:163-169, 1975.

20. Manual of the International Statistical Classification of Diseases, Injuries, and Causes of Death, 7th Revision Geneva: World Health Organisation, 1955.

21. Moses M, Selikoff IJ: Soft-tissue sarcoma, phenoxy herbicides, and chlorinated phenols. Lancet 1:1370, 1981.

22. Hardell L, Sandstrom A: Case-control study: Soft tissue sarcomas and exposure to phenoxyacetic acids or chlorophenols. Br J Cancer 39:711-717, 1979.

23. Ericksson M, Hardell L, Berg NO, Moller T, Axelson O: Soft-tissue sarcomas and exposure to chemical substances: A case-referent study. Br J Ind Med 38:27-33, 1981.

24. Smith AH, Pearce NE, Fisher DO, Giles HJ, Teague CA, Howard JK: Soft tissue sarcoma and exposure to phenoxyherbicides and chlorophenols in New Zealand. JNCI 73:1111-1117, 1984.

25. Cantor KP: Farming and mortality from non-Hodgkin's lymphoma: A case-control study. Int J Cancer 29:239-247, 1982.

26. Burmeister LF, Everett GD, Van Lier SF, Isacson P: Selected cancer mortality and farm practices in Iowa. Am J Epidemiol 118:72-77, 1983.

27. Fasal E, Jackson EW, Klauber MR: Leukemia and lymphoma mortality and farm residence. Am J Epidemiol 87:267-274, 1968.

28. Hardell L, Eriksson M, Lenner P, Lundgren E: Malignant lymphoma and exposure to chemicals, especially organic solvents, chlorophenols and phenoxy acids: A case-control study. Br J Cancer 43:169-176, 1981.

29. Markovitz A, Crosby WH: Chemical carcinogenesis: A soil fumigant, 1,3 - Dichloropropene, as possible cause of hematologic malignancies. Arch Intern Med 144:1409-1411, 1984.

30. Williams RR, Stegens NL, Goldsmith JR: Associations of cancer
     site and type with occupation and industry from the Third
     National Cancer Survey Interview. JNCI 59:1147-1185, 1977.

31. Buesching DP, Wollstadt L: Cancer mortality among farmers.
     JNCI 72:503, 1984.

32. Blair A, Fraumeni JF: Geographic patterns of prostate cancer in
     the United States. JNCI 61:1379-1384, 1978.

5

Ethylene Dibromide Toxicity and Fatal Consequences

JOHN OSTERLOH

INTRODUCTION

Ethylene dibromide has been in the news recently, particularly as a contaminant of food products and grains. Concern over possible adverse health effects following consumption of this food is necessary. However, potentially greater risks are present in the handling of this chemical in the work place. I will present two cases of fatal EDB exposure to emphasize the acute consequences of its toxicity.

Background

EDB is used as a soil fumigant for nematodes and a post-harvest fumigant for citrus and grains. Eighty-five percent of the 150 million kilograms produced annually is used as a lead scavenger when added to leaded gasoline.

(1) Chemically, EDB is a reactive alkylator with two active sites.

(2) In vitro and in vivo studies show it is metabolized to bromoethanol, bromoacetaldehyde, mono and diglutathione conjugates, beta-hydroxyethyl glutathione (the major urinary excretion product), and free bromide.

(3) EDB results in glutathione depletion in vitro.

(4) Following oral dosage in mice and guinea pigs, 12% of the dose is recovered in the expired air and 65% is excreted as metabolites in the urine and feces. The biological excretion half-life is 48 hours

(5) Complete recovery of radiolabelled EDB has not been shown in animal studies. This is possibly due to demonstrated reactions with other tissue sites including alkylation of DNA and protein. While EDB can directly react with DNA and protein, bromoethanol or bromoacetaldehyde metabolites are thought to be more reactive in this regard.

(6) Following 15 mg/kg oral single feedings of 14C-EDB, highest radioactivity is found in the liver > kidneys, > spleen, > testes = brain = fat at 24 hours after the dose.

Ethylene dibromide produces acute toxicity and has an LD50 of 55-420 mg/kg in various species. Following single acute pulmonary exposures, CNS depression and pulmonary hemorrhage may be observed. Application to the skin produces edema and necrosis of the skin. Following oral doses in animals, multiple organ necrosis is observed, particularly of the kidney and liver.

Ethylene dibromide is carcinogenic and produces gastric carcinomas in experimental animals after oral feedings. Hemangiosarcomas of the spleen and renal tumors have also been observed in chronic feeding studies. Ethylene dibromide is directly mutagenic in Ames type assays and mutagenic to Drosophila.

Bromoacetaldehyde and bromoethanol are also mutagenic. Ethylene dibromide is considered a reproductive hazard. It produces decreased egg production and egg weight in hens, abnormal sperm and sperm counts in bulls, and decreased litter size in rats.

Man is exposed during synthesis, formulation, shipping and fumigation, usually via respiratory or dermal routes. Respiratory and skin protection are mandatory. The new Cal-OSHA TLV of 130 ppb (1982) makes protecting the worker much more difficult. The previous TLV of 20 ppm was not considered protective against acute or potential longterm effects. The two cases that I will present occurred primarily due to lack of safety practices for which the formulating company received 17 citations by Cal-OSHA in 1982.

CASE 1.

A 31 year old male worker collapsed 5 minutes after entering a 7,500 gallon nurse tank following an attempt to clean its interior with pressurized water. He entered the tank with no respiratory or closed space precautions. Shortly after this, Case 2 entered the tank to rescue Case 1. Forty-five

minutes later, firefighters equipped with self-
contained breathing apparatus rescued both workers.
Case 1 was intermittently comatose, vomiting,
coughing and had burning of his eyes and throat. He
had a strong chemical odor, bothersome to his
rescuers. In the emergency room it was learned that
ethylene dibromide might have been the agent in the
tank. An admission bromide level later returned was
830 mg/L (endogenous = < 8 mg/L). At this time he was
slightly tachycardic and acidotic.

Because of anticipated respiratory chemical burns he
was transferred to a burn center. The helicopter
pilot complained of his chemical odor. Nearly 6
hours following the exposure, the patient was
semicomatose and in severe metabolic acidosis with
enzyme evidence of tissue injury (LDH, AST, CK were
elevated). His metabolic acidosis was treated with
90 meq IV bicarbonate, but was never satisfactorily
resolved. At 12 hours following the exposure, the
patient suffered a cardiopulmonary arrest and was not
able to be resuscitated.

CASE 2

The 46 year old supervisor who attempted to rescue
Case 1 was rescued by the firefighters after 20-30
minutes within the tank. At the scene, he was
delirious, combative, vomiting, and had complained of
burning eyes. At one hour he had regained his
consciousness and was coherent. He complained of
abdominal cramps and had a slight metabolic acidosis
and an elevated serum bromide level on presentation
to the hospital. He also had a strong chemical odor.

By 24 hours, dermal erythema and blisters had
appeared on his trunk and legs and oliguric renal
failure ensued. Again, evidence of tissue injury was
demonstrated by elevated serum enzyme levels. His
respiratory status was satisfactory in that partial
pressure of oxygen on room air was greater than 80
torr. His metabolic acidosis continued to worsen
over the next day and was twice treated with sodium
acetate hemodialysis. Following each hemodialysis
treatment, his blood pH would again quickly decrease.
At 64 hours, the patient suffered asystole and could
not be resuscitated.

The autopsy results in Case 1 showed passive
congestion of the viscera and the brain, bilateral
pulmonary edema and extensive multiorgan autolysis.
Autolysis was greater in the kidney and liver.

The post mortem findings in Case 2 showed extensive

advanced putrefaction. Most tissues showed autolysis
with an overgrowth of putrefactive organisms,
possibly enhanced by EDB damage. Grossly, the skin
showed blistering, desquamation and erythema in
exposed areas. Tissue bromides were measured in Case
2 and varied from 8-248 mg/L in various tissues with
highest levels in liver, kidney and spleen. The
ethylene dibromide was measurable in fat, thoracic
skin, leg skin and the brain. The sensitivity limit
of the assay was 0.5 ug/gm. EDB was not detected in
the heart, liver, lung, spleen or kidney. It is
thought that since metabolism may occur in these
tissues as opposed to fatty tissues, lesser
concentrations of the parent EDB would be found.

Tank analysis by Cal-OSHA the next day showed that
ethylene dibromide was in fact present in the three
inches of fluid at the tank bottom (0.1-0.3%). EDB
concentrations in the air may not have been
representative of EDB concentrations at the time of
exposure due to increased volatility from mist
formation by the pressurized water hose, and it would
not be expected that such concentrations would
acutely overcome an individual. The presence of
other gases or lack of oxygen in the tank (at the
time of the accident) had not been ruled out
analytically.

        The formulation plant site was observed by Cal-
OSHA to be an "unbelievably sloppy operation." The
operation was cited for 1) failure to train employees
in work practices, 2) failure to monitor airborne
concentrations of ethylene dibromide, 3) failure to
establish controls to reduce overexposure, 4) failure
to use proper respiratory protective equipment, 5)
failure to post precautionary signs, 6) failure to
have written confined-space operating procedures, 7)
failure to test and purge a confined space before
entering it, 8) failure to have employees wear
harness and safety belt when entering and working in
a confined space.

These two cases represent not only a tragic workplace
exposure, but possible exposure to all persons
involved directly with these two cases. Rescuers,
ambulance attendants, medical personnel, the
helicopter pilot, and pathologists, all
complained of a chemical odor. Even at autopsy,
several ppb of EDB in air was measured.

REFERENCES

1. Letz GA, Pond SM, Osterloh JD, Wade RL and Becker
   CE: Two fatalities after an acute occupational
   exposure to ethylene dibromide. JAMA 252:
   2428-2431, 1984.

6

PCB Risks in Fires, Accidents, and the Printing Industry: Part B—Risk Estimation and Application to PCB Fires and Printing Inks

JAMES E. CONE

INTRODUCTION

In the New York Times, on Friday December 7 an article entitled "Risks and Benefits, Disaster in India spreads net of fear and raises issue of technology's cost" analyzed that catastrophe in psychological terms. "The many hundreds of lives lost... were the result of a catastrophe that confirmed one's worst fears: that somewhere, perhaps everywhere, there are silent invisible man-made killers, from radiation, to gas, to asbestos" (1). And I would add, PCB's.

Dr. Marcel LaFollette, editor of Science, Technology and Human Values, was quoted in the same article, saying "We can build the technology, we can build the safeguards. We can even calculate the risks. But we cannot predict people's reactions based on emotion or lack of education or incompetence. There's always that unpredictable human factor" (1).

Risk benefit analysis has been developed to weigh the possible harm of a technology against economic and other possible benefits to society. However, as this article concludes, a problem with risk analysis is that it " reduces personal survival to a statistic. At best, it tries to decide what chance of tragedy is acceptable" (1).

Today, I will discuss the case of PCB's in fires and in printing ink, to address this question: Is risk analysis of any use in such situations to answer the question, not just what risk we face from future potential exposures to buildings contaminated in the past with PCB's, but what risk is there from past exposure for those who were there and unknowingly exposed.

I.   Principles of Risk Assessment:

Some form of risk estimation has long been used by
toxicologists to evaluate toxic exposures situations.   In
the traditional form, at least since the 1950's, two steps
were outlined: (2)

1.   An extrapolation to low level exposures using data
from high dose carcinogenesis assay was performed. A dose
which corresponded to a given lifetime cancer risk was
then calculated.

2.   An acceptable daily intake was established based on a
"no observed effect level (NOEL)".

However, this traditional approach has been challenged due
to the restriction from FDA that an Acceptable Daily
Intake (ADI) cannot be extrapolated from a NOEL for
compounds that have been found to be carcinogenic.

Some exception to this has been made for compounds found
not to be genotoxic. The justification for this has not
been clearly outlined, however.
More recently, Bob Tardiff has outlined a four-step
conceptual basis for Risk Assessment: (3)

STEP I: Hazard Identification and Evaluation.

The review and evaluation of various types of experimental
and epidemiological data to identify the **qualitative**
nature of the hazards associated with a substance or
activity. The questions include whether a substance is a
carcinogen, and the strength of the evidence. Other acute
or chronic toxicity, such as neurotoxicity, reproductive
toxicity, or respiratory toxicity are also identified.

STEP II: The Dose-response evaluation.

The quantitative relationship between exposure and risk is
estimated and then extrapolated from the conditions of
exposure for which data exist to   other conditions of
interest.   This assumes that the dose-response
relationship does not disappear   at the detection limit
of exposure or epidemiologic investigation.

This also assumes that a biologically plausible model for
the characteristics of the dose response curve exists and
makes assumptions about the quantitative relationship
between the test animal dose and response function, and
those applied to human populations.

STEP III: Identification of the conditions of exposure:

This step first involves evaluation of the **intensity** of
exposure,   usually involving industrial hygiene
measurements of the exposure level by the various
potential routes of exposure.
Second, an evaluation of the **frequency** potential future
exposure (eg. days per week or year of of expected
exposure) is made.

The third condition of exposure, the total average
expected **duration** of exposure (eg working life of 30 yrs.)
is then estimated for the population.

The final condition of exposure involves assumptions about
the characteristics of the population of interest, for
example height or weight of the standard person expected
to be exposed (eg 50 kg
65 inch tall female, or 70 kg. male with average height
of 70 inches).

STEP IV: The Probability of the Hazard.

Thus, risk assessment, according to Tardiff, involves the
combination of the dose- with response, leading to an
estimated probability that the hazards associated with a
substance or activity will be seen under the conditions of
exposure experienced by the population at risk.

B.   Risk Management:

Tardiff separates this from Risk Assessment per se.   This
enters the realm of policy, and involves the decision
whether the assessed risk is important or not.

The magnitude of the risk is estimated, and degree of
confidence in the data is assessed.   Some estimation of
the strength of the evidence supporting the position that
the substance is hazardous is key. An estimate is made of
the extent of variability of risk under different
assumptions and models.

In the past, risk assessment has been largely applied to
future and potential exposures, attempting to set a level
of risk which is "acceptable" to society, or as the NY
Times article puts it, the "level of tragedy which is
acceptable" (1), and may result in standard setting.

However, occupational health professionals are often in a
position of responding to existing exposures or prior
relatively uncontrolled exposures, and are asked to
estimate probabilities of risk for future events such as
cancer.

Although not generally used in past risk estimations, I
will attempt to extend the application of risk analysis
to estimate risks of populations already exposed. This
retrospective risk analysis attempts to reconstruct an
individual's exposure, and compare this with levels of
exposure which have been found in animal studies to be
lead to observable increases in cancer. This then is more
of a qualitative risk assessment, to answer the question:
Was I exposed to a dose which could cause cancer in the
future?

This approach may then involve choosing biological
monitoring tools which then may be used to estimate
absorbed dose (eg. PCB serum levels, fat TCDD levels). A
decision then must be made whether the biological
monitoring tools confirm the estimated exposure level, or
not.

II. CASE STUDY FROM PREVIOUS PCB FIRE IN BINGHAMPTON, NY

The first application of risk assessment methods to TCDD's
was performed by EPA's Carcinogen Assessment Group in 1980
(cited in 2). Using a carcinogenic extrapolation
procedure, they came up with a 1 in a million "acceptable
risk level" corresponding with a dose of 2.36×10^{-9}
ug/kg-day.

The risk assessment process at a previous PCB fire at
Binghampton, New York state office building is instructive
as an example of the application of this process (2).

There, a fire caused by malfunctioning PCB-containing
transformer on February 6, 1981 released a soot-like
material containing incomplete combustion products
including 2,3,7,8-TCDD, TCDF's and high concentrations of
numerous other isomers, along with the PCB into the 18
story building.

The risk estimate was developed to set a standard for
cleanup of the building before reentry. Analyzing this
risk assessment process using the steps outlined by
Tardiff:

1. Hazard identification and evaluation: The NYSHD
performed toxicological and animal studies on the soot
obtained from the building. They took results of previous
studies on TCDD to make the initial assessment that TCDD
is in fact a carcinogen, with multiple other potential
toxic effects seen at higher exposure levels, but state
that it is not a genotoxin based on the studies reviewed.

As an aside, I would question this assumption, since
studies of repeated or single doses of TCDD in mice, show

that as little as 1 ug/kg resulted in increased
frequencies of cleft palate and kidney abnormalities in
offspring (5) , and in rats (6).

The lethal dose for 50 percent of test animals from TCDD
runs from microgram to miligrams for various species.
Other chronic effects (weight loss, lymphoid atrophy,
chloracne, hair loss, porphyria, and enzyme induction)
may be seen in the nanogram range. (7)

II. The dose-response evaluation was based on a key
assumption that TCDD was the most toxic agent present in
the soot, and that chronic TCDD data could be used as a
basis for the dose-response evaluation.   A NOEL was
assumed based on a TCDD NOEL of 1 ng/kg-day in rats seen
in a three generation reproduction study (3) and a two
year cancer study (4). An "uncertainty factor" was used
to extrapolate to humans, intitially 100, and later 500.
The selection of an uncertainty factor of 100 was
initially justified by citing long-term animal studies.
Later, the Expert Advisory Panel set up for the risk
assessment changed this to 500. This is obviously a key
area of imprecision in the risk assessment process, with
dramatic effects on the eventual level arrived at. Using
this uncertainty factor, a daily total dose of 2 pg/kg-day
was arrived at.

III. The conditions of exposure were assumed to fit the
following: Exposure primarily through inhalation, but
also through dermal absorbtion and ingestion, assuming 30
year exposure, 250 working days/year, and 10 cubic meter
respiratory volume per working day.   The typical building
inhabitant was assumed to be a 50 kg female.

Three different scenarios of environmental decay were
examined: I. assuming daily exposure were constant over
the 30 years, II. Contamination levels declined to 1% of
initial value over 30 years, and III. 1st order
decontamination curve with t1/2 of 1 year.

The total exposure limit for the 50 kg female was thus 2
pg/kg-day X 50 = 100 pg/day. An air level was thus set,
assuming all exposure through the air, of 10 pg/m3 of
TCDD. Using the acute toxicity equivalent of the soot
(ratio of soot/TCDD) of 58/1.2, a air soot level of 10
pg/m3 X 58/1.2 = 483 pg/m3 of soot was obtained.
Similarly, a PCDF level was estimated.

Surface area guidelines were set by assuming surface area
of the average female, with a certain percentage exposed
(hands and arms), and absorbtion of 1% -10%, resulting in
a range of 3 ng/m2 to 28 ng/m2 surface contamination
standard for TCDD.

IV.   The probability of the hazard

A risk management level was implicit in the Risk
Assessment, set such that the risk of additional case of
cancer among future exposed was 1/10⁶.

III.   CASE STUDIES FROM THE OCCUPATIONAL HEALTH CLINIC,
SFGH

1.   One Market St. PCB Transformer Fire

   The first situation we faced at the Occupational Health
Clinic, San Francisco General Hospital which required the
use of the tools of risk estimation was the 1 Market Plaza
PCB fire.

Subsequent to the fire, a risk assessment procedure was
undertaken by the Epidemiologic Studies Section,
California State Department of Health Services.   (8)

This procedure followed similar asssumptions and process
as the Binghampton Risk Assessment (2).   The differences
with Binghampton were the following: The risk management
level was set such that no additional cases of cancer
would be expected to occur given a 40 year exposure. A
second principle was established, that even though a small
exposed population might not be expected to develop an
extra case of cancer, the individuals in that group should
not have to accept an unreasonable actuarial risk of
additional cancer.   Theoretical   risks were set at 1/10⁶.
Again, a 500 fold safety factor for chronic and
reproductive effects was used, a 15,000 fold   safety
factor for embryotoxic effects and a 50,000 fold factor
for teratogenic effects, again based on a NOEL for TCDD in
animals.   An additional factor is mentioned: the ability
to accurately measure such a level in a reasonable number
of samples.

Finally, they recommend comparison inspections of other
similar office buildings to set a background level.

The recommended standard for cleanup was set at 10 pg/m3
of TCDD/TCDF in air inside the building, and an 80 pg/m3
level in the actual vault of the transformer, assuming
that it is visited only 2 hours a month.

However, we at the Occupational Health Clinic were faced
with the questions of passerbys, newsmedia, building
maintenance and firefighters about the level of risk they
had encumbered as a result of their individual exposures.
We were not able to give a precise estimation at the time,
which then prompted us to try to develop more of a
quantitative risk estimation method for both this fire and
the similar   future episodes which may   occur.

STEP I.   Hazard Identification and Evaluation.

The 1 Market St. Fire occurred on May 15, 1983, during the largest footrace in the world, the Bay to Breakers. Dr. Letz has outlined the literature on the known hazards of PCB's, TCDF's and TCDD's.   Using the same analysis and assumptions as the prospective risk assessment, we assume that the most toxic material present in the smoke and soot was TCDD/TCDF, with carcinogenic risks as outlined.

STEP II.   Dose-response evaluation.
Animal studies looking at cancer outcomes from one-time doses or short-term exposures are lacking.   Thus we are forced to extrapolate from chronic feeding studies to short-term inhalation type exposures.   From such feeding studies, 1 ng/kg-wk of TCDD was the lowest dose without observed increase in neoplasms (5).

No no-effect level for carcinogens such as TCDD is assumed.   A 500-fold safety factor is desirable in extrapolation between species.

STEP III: Identification of the conditions of exposure.

Here, we were relied on extensive industrial hygiene evaluations performed by Richard Wade, consultant industrial hygienist for the City and County of San Francisco (9),   and statements by the exposed persons themselves about the duration and nature of their exposure and protective equipment worn.   The areas of the building involved were categorized by zone, assuming similar exposure levels within each zone.

TABLE 1:

Average Exposure levels (surface wipe samples)
by zone at the time of the 1 Mkt. St. PCB fire (9)
5/15/83

Zone #	Description	PCB ug/100 cm°2	TCDF ng/m°2
1	Inside Vault and directly in smoke standing on top of vault cover on sidewalk	300,000	15,600
2.	Soot and fumes less than 50 feet from vault cover on sidewalk	16,000	–
3.	Inside switchgear room, on Basement (B2) and in woodshop (Basement B1)	40-50	–
4.	Inside fan room	20-30	–
5.	Outside perimeter (50-200 ft. from vault cover)	1.4	ND
6.	Inside stairwells including freight elevator	3-4	–
7.	Inside Lobby area near high rise elevators, and in parking lot	1.0	–
8.	Zone more than 200 ft from vault cover and all other external sites	0	–

The duration of exposure varied from 15 minutes to 3 hours during the actual fire itself (until the power could be shut off), and from less than 1 hour to over 100 hours for persons involved in initial stages of cleanup and evaluation. Direct contact with smoke was reported by 108/162 of the persons who volunteered to be evaluated by a screening medical questionnaire at the SFGH Occupational Health Clinic, and soot was noted on the clothing in 89 (55%). Soot was noted to be present on hands, face or skin by 58 or 35%. During the initial period, protective clothing, including double boots, double gloves, Air supplied respirator, hood and tyvek suit were worn **only** by persons who entered the vault area. One person, an electric company employee, reportedly did enter the vault without such protective equipment, for a total of a few minutes.

IV. Probability of hazard

To answer the question raised by many of those exposed, regarding possible future health risk due to their exposure, we attempted to assess the duration of exposure, whether it was to the fire or cleanup, location of exposure, dermal vs. respiratory route, and use of protective equipment to develop an exposure index for the participants in the survey. Missing, and impossible to answer at this time is the expected latency for any health effects including cancer resulting from a single or short-term exposure.

Example I. The Electric Company Employee.

One of the most highly exposed individuals, the electric company employee, most likely had a short term exposure to soot containing 300,000 ug/100 cm2 of PCB, and 15,600 ng/m2 of TCDF. He did not participate in the OHC surveillance program, but we estimated his total exposure, based on a presumed body weight of 70 kg., and a total exposure time of 15 minutes, with respiratory volume of 7 cubic meters over 8 hours X .25 hours = .2 cubic meters. Dermal exposure calculations assumed a total body surface area of $7.184 \times 10^{\circ}-3 \times wt^{\circ}.425 \times height^{\circ}.725 = 1.91$ square meters. Dermal exposure on arms (20% of total body surface area), with 10 percent absorbtion, was thus equivalent to a surface area of 0.0191 square meters. Oral exposure is assumed to be non-contributory. Thus an estimated total dose to this individual would be his respiratory dose (unmeasured at the time of the fire but probably considerable as well), plus his dermal exposure (0.0191 m2 X 300,000 ug/100 cm2 X 100 =573000 ug or 573 mg of PCB, and 0.0191 m2 X 15,600 ng/m2 = 298 ng of TCDF.

Thus, this dose of dermal exposure alone is equivalent to
298/70 = 4.25 times the lowest equivalent weekly TCDD dose
without carcinogenic effect in chronic animal studies, and
presumably, the respiratory dose would have been
relatively high as well, increasing this estimate
somewhat.

Example 2:   Building Maintenance Worker.

A second example is one of the maintenance workers who had
both an acute exposure on the day of the fire for several
hours, including smoke exposure, as well as various types
of chronic exposure to contaminated areas of the building
over a period of weeks.

We chronicled his exposure times and locations, to attempt
to arrive at a total dose of exposure:

DAY of FIRE:

1.   Switch Gear room, entered 6 times, 10 minutes each for
total of 60 minutes. Air levels later measured to be 300-
700 ug/m3, and floor of room 58 ug/100 cm2.   Total
exposure:

(AIR) =   7/8 m3 air/1 hr. X 700 ug/m3 = 612 ug   PCB

+   (SKIN) =   0.0191 m2 X 58 ug/100 cm2   X 10000 = 11,078
ug PCB

2.   Fan room, entered 6 times, 15 minutes each for a total
of 90 minutes. Air levels were 70-90 ug/m3, and surfaces
with 20-30 ug/100 cm2.   Total exposure:

AIR = 1.3 m3 air /1.5 hr X 90 ug/m3 = 117 ug PCB
SKIN= 0.0191 m2 X 30 ug/100 cm2 X 10000 =   5730 ug PCB

3. Woodshop, briefly the day of the fire, dermal exposure
only:

SKIN = 0.0191 m2 X 3000 ug/100 cm2 X 10000 = 573000 ug
PCB.

Thus, the day of the fire, a conservative estimate of
total absorbtion of PCB's would be 590,537 ug PCB.

He then worked for four days following the fire, totalling
70 hours, without protective gear, since the TCDF
contamination was not yet known. He spent a total of 4
hours in the switch gear room, 8 hours in the fan room, 16
hours in woodshop. Using estimates derived similarly to
the above calculations, and multiplying only by the air
level timed exposures, and adding an equivalent daily skin
exposure, the total from these four days is:

```
Switch gear room 2400 + 44000  =        46,400 ug  PCB
Fan room 624 + 22920           =        23,544 ug  PCB
Woodshop                       =     2,000,000 ug  PCB
                                     ------------------
                                     2,069,944 ug  PCB
```

Following notification of contamination, he no longer
entered these areas, but he then ate lunch daily in
another area directly above the vault for 23 days, total
of 1 hour daily. This area was subsequently found to have
up to 3000 ug/100 cm2 of PCB on surfaces. Total of
exposure (SKIN) = 573000 ug/day PCB. X 23 days =
12,029,000 ug PCB = 12 gm of PCB.

He then was notified of this exposure, and then spent the
following two weeks in complete personal protective
equipment, with tyvek suit, respirator, etc., 3 hours/day
in first week, and 1.5 hours/day in second week in
woodshop area. Assuming a 10,000:1 protection factor of
this Personal Protective Equipment, his exposure then
would be:

5.7 ug PCB/day X 14 days = 79 ug PCB dermal only.

A total TCDF dose may then be estimated. First, a ratio
of 20 ug of PCB to 1 ng of TCDF was observed in locations
where simultaneous analysis for both substances was
performed. If this is is assumed to be true over this
maintenance worker's total exposure, then this represents
an exposure total to TCDF of 14,689,000 ug /20 = 734,000
ng of TCDF, or 734 ug TCDF over a 5 week period.

He was evaluated about 2 months later for this exposure
and had a measurement of serum total PCB of < 5 ppb, and
fat total PCB of < 200 ppb. He also at that time had a
chest x-ray showing a lung nodule, which was subsequently
shown to be a squamous cell carcinoma on pathology at
resection.

The questions raised by this example include the
following:

What effect did his extensive exposure to PCB (and PCDF)
have on the development of this tumor, detected only 2
months later? Why, after the extensive reported
exposure, did his serum and fat biopsy show low level of
PCB? What would his expected risk of another carcinoma
be, given his estimated exposure level, which is many
times the lowest chronic animal dose which produced
carinomas?

A third example at the opposite extreme of exposure is
that of a passerby who was in the smoke for 5 minutes, who
noticed visable black soot on hands and arms. Assuming
that the exposure is equivalent to zone 2, with 16,000
ug/cm2 surface contamination, and again, air levels not
determined, dermal exposure alone could be estimated. For
a 70 kg male, the absorbed dose of such an exposure to
skin would be: 0.0191 m2 X 16000 ug/100 cm2 X 10000 =
3,056,000 ug absorbed PCB, or 152,800 ng of PCDF's.

Thus, in light of the demonstrated presence of PCDF's in
addition to PCB's, and the potential dose levels which
could be estimated based on industrial hygiene
measurements performed shortly after the fire, a large
proportion of the population exposed to this fire,
including passerbys as well as firefighters and building
maintenance workers most likely did have significant
exposures to both PCB's and PCDF's, and may incur
increased risk of long term health effects in the future.
The latency of such health effects is difficult to
predict based on existing knowledge.

SITUATION II: PCB Contamination of Printing Inks:

In January, 1984, a sample of yellow newspaper ink used
for color printing at a local newspaper was found to
contain a quantitly of a single isomer of PCB, 3,3'
dichlorobiphenyl. Later samples of the same yellow ink
were analyzed and found to have between 6 ppm and 4,100
ppm of this isomer.

The State Department of Health Services was asked to
perform a toxicological review of literature on this and
similar compounds. This review was performed by John
Rosenberg (10). The 3,3' DCBP was formed as a side
reaction in the manufacture of Pigment Yellow 12 from 3,3'
dichlorobenzidine. It was hypothesized that the reaction
forming the 3,3' DCBP took place at the end of the
manufacturing process to deaminate any residual
dichlorobenzidine due to concern over the carcinogenicity
of DCB.

Workers were exposed to various concentrations of this
PCB, from manufacture of pigment, formulation of
concentrated pigment, dilution of the concentrate, and use
as ink.

A risk assessment of this exposure using the methods
outlined above will be performed:

I.   Hazard Identification and Evaluation:

HESIS, in its toxicology review (10), noted that
toxicology studies of any isomers of dichlorobiphenyl are
almost entirely lacking. Pure isomers are difficult to

produce, and most commercial PCB's are mixtures, with only
a small fraction of them with diclorobiphenyls.

The toxicity of PCB isomers was noted to be correlated
with the isomer's ability to induce Aryl Hydrocarbon
hydroxylase (AHH) or P448 system in the liver, and depend
on the degree and position of chlorination.

The dichlorobiphenyls have been tested, including 3,3'-
DCBP, for AHH induction ability (10) and 3,3' was found to
be completely inactive at a dose where Arochlor 1260
produced marked induction.

The toxicity of this isomer, by this method, was expected
to be relatively low.

Other studies were reviewed, including studies of 4,4'
DCBP, showing that metabolism was rapid, with t1/2 of 1
day for excretion in dogs. It was predicted that if this
was true for 3,3' as well, it would be rapidly excreted,
and little accumulated. The metabolism process involves
converting the fat soluble PCB into a water-soluble
hydroxylated molecule which then is excreted in the urine.
This process, however, is performed via an arene oxide
intermediate, and arene oxide intermediates have been
linked to carcinogenicity due to their binding to cellular
macromolecules. Levinskas, in his review of PCB's and
carcinogenicity, states that "taken as a whole, metabolism
studies suggest that if PCB's are carcinogenic, it should
be those PCB's which are more readily metabilized and
excreted, ie the lower chlorinated materials." (13)
However, as he points out, these conclusions drawn from
metabolism studies are not supported by the animal data,
which support the opposite conclusion.

Thus, on balance, the 3,3' dichlorobiphenyl isomer would
be expected to have low relative acute toxicity, and the
carcinogenic potential would also be judged to be low,
based on animal feeding studies.

STEP II. Dose response evaluation. Due to the lack of
animal studies of carcinogenicity of this isomer, it is
impossible to undertake a dose-response evaluation.

STEP III. Identification of the conditions of exposure:

The intensity of exposure was measured by industrial
hygienists from CAL/OSHA. Bulk samples of ink measured
from 58-4100 ppm depending on use. Samples were also
analyzed for dichlorobenzidine, and found to have less
than 20 ppm. Since this was a pigment, not a dye, it was
felt by the industrial hygienist to be relatively
insoluble, thus reducing the toxicity.

Analysis for TCDD or TCDF were not performed, since these were not expected to be byproducts of the manufacturing process.

Air samples were below the detection limit of 3 ug/m3. Wipe samples were obtained, due to the potential considerable contact that pressmen may have with the printing ink. Results ranged from 0.2 ug/100 cm2 to 3.1 ug/100 cm2. Bulk samples of ink inside of presses had a maximum of 100 ppm. (14)

Frequency of past exposure was judged to be daily, for an indeterminate period, at least for 6 months prior to discovery of the contamination.

Thus, using the methods of estimating dose illustrated previosly,
the dose of 3,3'-DCBP which would be expected to have been absorbed by the average pressman who worked 5 days/wk, 8 hrs./day for 6 months at the upper limit of exposure levels measured (assuming that any measurement below the detection limit would be at that limit) would equal:

Airborne: 7 m3/day X 3 ug/m3 X 120 days = 2550 ug.
 In terms of daily dose/kg = 21 mg/70kg = .3 ug/kg-day

Dermal: 0.0191 m2 X 3.1 ug/100 cm2 x 10000 X 120 days = 71052 ug. In terms of daily dose/kg = 8 ug/kg-day.

TOTAL: 73,602 ug. 3,3' DCBP. (8.3 ug/kg-day)

This compares with chronic rat feeding studies with Arochlor 1260 and 1254 which showed adenofibrosis of liver beginning at about 7 mg/kg-day, or roughly 1000 times greater daily intake.

IV. The probability of the hazard

A medical monitoring program was undertaken by us at the OHC, SFGH, to determine if there were detectable acute or chronic health effects of such exposures. We also attempted to document the extent of exposure using biological monitoring, in this case, serum and fat PCB levels.

The serum total PCB levels were undetectable, with detection limit of 5 ppb, in all but two workers who had 10 ppb in serum. This is well within the range seen in non-occupationally exposed populations (up to 30 ppb).

Total fat PCB levels ranged from 234 ppb to 1624 ppb, with a mean of 650 ppb. Again, this is well below the usual upper limit of non-occupationally exposed persons reported in the literature. Isomer specific levels are pending.

We thus concluded that at the exposure levels which we could document, and with the levels of total PCB seen on fat biopsy, we did not predict that pressmen exposed to 3,3' DCBP would have significantly increased risk of developing long term health effects from this exposure in the future.

SUMMARY AND CONCLUSIONS:

Thus, using two examples of the application of risk estimation to prior exposures, I hopefully have illustrated some of the usefulness as well as the imprecision and difficulties:

1. Usefulness

A qualitative answer to the question of whether increased risk of future health effects after known exposure to PCB's may be given, qualified by the uncertainty of extrapolation from limited animal data, and imprecision of exposure data.

2. Difficulties

1. Imprecise exposure data -- difficult to project back in time to period of actual exposure.

2. Lacking animal data on exact exposure of interest: eg. soot or smoke in fires, which vary depending on isomers and contaminants of PCB's present, or exact isomers of PCB in ink.

3. Lacking confirmation of respiratory and dermal absorbtion rates in varying conditions.

4. This raises the issue of what to do with information: Should PCB fire victims be enrolled in an exposure registry and followed for possible development of cancer over their lifetime? What should be done to deal with the anxiety raised by the suspicion of significant dose of a known carcinogen?

5. Most importantly, this analysis supports the position that PCB-containing transformers and capacitors must be replaced immediately to reduce the potential risks of further episodes.

FUTURE ISSUES:

1. How many of the future cancers in PCB fire exposed persons will be attributable to the fire?

2. If PCB's are in fact promoters rather than initiators of carcinogensis as some would argue, how does this affect our risk estimate?

REFERENCES CITED

(1)   Broad WJ. Risks and benefits: disaster in India
       spreads net of fear and raises issue of technology's
       cost. New York Times, Friday December 7, 1984, p. 10.
(2)   Kim N. Revised Risk Estimation, Binghamptom State
       Office Building. June 7, 1983 Draft.
(3)   Rodricks JD and Tardiff RG. Conceptual basis for risk
       assessment.   In Rodricks JD and Tardiff RG, eds.
       Assessment and management of chemical risks. ACS
       Symposium Series 239. American Chemical Society,
       Washington,D.C., 1984.
(4)   Murray FJ, et al. Three generation reproduction
       study of rats given 2,3,7,8 TCDD in the diet.
       Toxicology and App. Pharm. 1979;50:241-52.
(5)   Kociba RJ, et. al., Results of a two-year chronic
       toxicity and oncogenicity study of 2,3,7,8-TCDD in
       rats.   Toxicology and App. Pharm. 1978;46:279-303.
(6)   Courtney KD, Moore JA, Teratology studies Iwith
       2,4,5-T and TCDD. Arch. Exptl. Pathol. Pharmakol.
       1972;272:243, cited in (7).
(7)   Huff JE, et. al. Long term hazards of PCDD and PCDF.
       Env. Hlth. Perspectives 1980;36:221-40.
(8)   Gravitz N, et.al. Interim guidelines for acceptable
       exposure levels in office settings contaminated with
       PCB and PCB contamination products. Epidemiological
       Studies Section, California Department of Health
       Services, 2151 Berkeley Way, Berkeley CA 94704,
       September 30, 1983.
(9)   Richard Wade, Personal Communication.
(10)   Rosenberg J. Assessment of the hazard of 3,3' -
       Diclorobiphenyl in yellow newspaper ink. Hazard
       Evaluation System and Information Service, State of
       California, 2151 Berkeley Way, Berkeley CA 94704, May
       1984.
(11)   Silkworth J, et. al. Acute toxicity in guinea pigs
       and rabbits of soot from a polychlorinated Biphenyl
       containing transformer fire. Center for Laboratories
       and Research, NYSDH. Albany NY, Tox. Appl. Pharmacol.
       1982.
(12)   Goldstein JA, Chem. Biol. Interactions 1977;17:69-
       87.
(13)   Levinskas GJ. A review and evaluation of
       carcinogenicity studies in mice and rats and
       mutagenicity studies with polychlorinated biphenyls.
       Unpublished draft, October 14, 1981.
(14)   Tuse B. Survey Summary, San Jose Mercury News.
       CAL/OSHA, September 13, 1984.

7

Danger of Handling Oncological Agents

LUCI A. POWER

INTRODUCTION

The quality of the hospital environment, recently questioned in
light of worker exposure to ethylene oxide and anesthetic gases, is
once again under scrutiny due to current practices in the handling of
oncological agents.[1] Many of these agents are potent, and sometimes
toxic, chemicals. Several have been implicated in the development of
secondary cancers in patients who received therapeutic doses of these
agents during the treatment of a primary malignancy.[2]

The fact that many oncological agents are caustic and/or vesicants
that may cause immediate reactions in the health care personnel who
handle them is undisputed. The possibility that these drugs may
cause a greater occupational hazard, that of exposure to mutagens
and/or carcinogens, is under investigation.

RESEARCH

In 1979, Falck reported that nurses handling oncological, or
cytotoxic, agents had greater levels of mutagenicity, as measured by
the Ames test, in their urine than did controls not involved in the
care of cancer patients.[3] This finding was followed by several
anecdotal reports of unpleasant side effects suffered by nurses,
nursing students, pharmacists and pharmacy technicians while
preparing these agents.[4,5,]

In 1980, Melvyn Davis of Australia, using black background
photography with a high speed trigger, demonstrated drug particles
escaping into the environment from both ampuls and vials of
oncological agents. Kleinberg and Quinn at the University of
California, San Diego, validated Davis' findings with air sampling
of routine manipulation of ampuls and vials in a horizontal,
laminar-flow hood.[6] Neal, Wadden and Chiou at the University of
Illinois, Chicago, performed ambient-air sampling of four

oncological agents in ten outpatient oncology clinics.[7] Two of the
four drugs were detectable and identifiable by the methods selected
by the researchers. Since no safe level of occupational exposure to
these agents has been determined, it is impossible to state whether
the levels detected by either of the research methods were
"significant".

Sister chromatid exchange (SCE) has also been used to determine the
biological effects of oncological agents on nurses. Norppa et. al.
found an increased sister chromatid exchange frequency in
lymphocytes of nurses handling cytotoxic drugs.[8] Waksvik and co-
workers also found increased chromatid exchange frequencies and an
increased incidence of chromosome gaps in nurses handling
oncological agents for more than 2000 hours.[9] Both studies,
however, are subject to criticism and do not present definitive
evidence of occupational risk.

In 1982, Anderson et. al. published the results of a logitudinal
study of urine mutagenicity, as measured by the Ames test, in
pharmacy personnel who prepared oncological agents in horizontal
laminar-flow hoods.[10] Mutagenicity was observed in the urine of all
personnel during periods when they prepared the drugs, increasing as
the days of exposure increased. The Anderson study used 24 hour
urine collections, from each subject, over an eight-day period,
beginning after several day's absence from possible exposure. Three
strains of test organisms were used; all test organisms were not
sensitive in every test with each subject. Each subject exhibited a
unique pattern of mutagenic activity, with peaks occurring on days
5, 6, and 7 of the work week. No subject showed mutagenic activity,
defined as 2 times background, prior to 48 hours of exposure. No
mutagenicity was detected in the control group nor in the exposed
group when admixtures were prepared in a contained, vertical air
flow, biological safety cabinet.

Other studies using the Ames test were not supportive of the results
of Falck's or Anderson's studies. The National Institutes of Health
(NIH), in March, 1981, reported a lack of mutagenic activity, as
measured by the Ames test, in urine from hospital pharmacists
mixing oncological agents.[11] As designed, 24 hour samples were
collected two days before and at the time of exposure and 48 hours
thereafter. The failure of NIH to reproduce Falck's data may be due
to the selection of sampling days, which differed considerably from
the original study, and the fact that most of the subjects in the
NIH study were already protected by the use of a biological safety
cabinet during preparation.

In 1983, Sotaniemi et al published case reports of three nurses,
each of whom, after years of handling oncological agents, developed
liver damage.[12] Although the liver injury cannot be exclusively
linked to the occupational exposure, this finding is, nevertheless,
significant.

Of even greater significance is the work by researchers in Canada
who recently reported conclusive identification of cyclophosphamide
in several urine samples from nurses preparing and administering
that drug.[13] Similar research with platinum-containing drugs in
Great Britain failed to detect urinary platinum as markers of
absorption.[14] While the British study may appear to question the
Canadian results, the subjects in the British study used protective
garments, gloves and masks, during exposure, the Canadians did not.
The results of the British study, therefore, could indicate that
personal, protective garments are effective for handling platinum-
containing compounds safely.

Interpretation of the research published to date has lead to some
controversy regarding the significance of this possible occupational
hazard. A recent Lancet editorial stated the data thus far did not
substantiate costly safety measures while a rebuttal letter pointed
out that a conservative judgment should be on the side of safety
rather than short term economics.[15,16]

REGULATION

The Occupational Safety and Health Administration (OSHA), empowered
by the Federal government to protect employees, has cited hospitals
in the states of Missouri, South Carolina and Oklahoma for failure
to adequately protect health care workers who handle oncological
agents and has mandated effective occupational safety and health
programs for these employees.[17]

California is one of several states that administers its own
occupational safety and health program according to the provisions
of the federal Occupational Safety and Health Act of 1970. The
California Occupational Safety and Health Administration (Cal/OSHA)
has cited several hospitals where the methods of handling
oncological agents was considered by Cal/OSHA potentially
hazardous.[18]

In response to numerous requests for consultations, Cal/OSHA
published extensive recommendations directed at establishing safety
programs for the preparation and administration of parenteral
oncologics.[19]

The results of current research, taken as a whole, and regulatory
agency activity to date should be sufficient evidence to encourage
the prudent hospital and pharmacy administrator to develop
comprehensive safety programs based on the assessment of risks to
the workers in an individual institution.

PROTECTION

Once the risks have been assessed and a projected level of safety
determined, administrative controls, protective equipment and
engineering controls must be selected to attain that level. The

postulated routes of exposure for these agents are the same as for any occupational hazard: absorption through skin or other membranes, inhalation of powder or liquid aerosols, inadvertent ingestion of contaminated food or drink and the possibility of accidental injection while handling a contaminated needle or other sharp object. Safety measures, recommended to protect against these routes of exposure, are based on accepted theories of occupational safety and common sense.[20,21]

Engineering Controls

The use of engineering controls during the preparation of oncological agents is of primary importance. Engineering controls reduce the level of contamination in the environment, and subsequently in the worker, by containing the hazardous agent at its source and usually function independently of worker technique. Other protective systems increase the efficacy of engineering controls but require constant monitoring to ensure compliance.

The Class II, biological safety cabinet (BSC) has been recommended as an effective engineering control for the safe preparation of parenteral oncological agents.[20,21] As previously discussed, Anderson et al. demonstrated that installing a BSC in the preparation area reduced the levels of mutagenic substances detected in the urine of pharmacy workers preparing these agents.[10]

Protective Garments And Equipment

In addition to the BSC, workers preparing oncological agents should use proper barrier garments. A disposable, closed front, non-absorbent gown and good quality surgical latex gloves are suitable protection in handling most oncological agents. These garments are recommended to prevent body contact and subsequent contamination both during preparation and administration of these agents. The use of a BSC and barrier garments is standard practice in any laboratory where mutagenic and carcinogenic material is handled.

During preparation of oncological agents in the absence of a BSC, while administering them, cleaning up a spill or in any instance which could result in exposure by inhalation, respiratory protection is recommended. Inexpensive respirator masks are available to reduce inhalation of powder and liquid aerosols; standard surgical masks have limited effectiveness against inhalation of aerosols and are not recommended for this purpose.

Eye protection should always be used during preparation of any of the vesicants in a non-protected environment. Safety goggles or a plexiglass face shield are adequate protection against inadvertent eye damage. Gowns, double gloves, respirators and eye protection are recommended for use when cleaning up a spill of an oncological agent.

Technique

Meticulous aseptic technique is a must whenever these agents are prepared or administered. The amount of environmental contamination is directly dependent on the amount of drug allowed to escape into the air. Avoid pressurizing vials during reconstitution and withdrawal of drug. This reduces "blow back" of the drug from the vial top. Sterile gauze should be used to cover vial tops, ampuls and needles to prevent drug from leaking or spraying into the environment. When measuring drug or priming IV lines, excess drug should be discarded onto absorbent material that is quickly sealed into air-tight containers.

Many devices are currently available that make handling vials and ampuls of oncological agent safer and more efficient. Long "filter straws" may be used with ampuls to allow removal of the drug while holding the ampul upright. The "straw" prevents the glass from passing into the syringe and cannot be used for injecting the drug into a line, bottle or bag.

Adding or withdrawing from a closed vial has been made easier by the use of vented needles or pins that equilibrate the pressures inside and outside of the closed system. Special venting devices have been designed to work with oncological agents. These devices have a 0.22 micron hydrophobic membrane filter attached to the venting pathway. Powder or liquid aerosols are trapped on the filter preventing contamination of the atmosphere. As with all devices, practice is imperative to ensure proper and effective operating technique.

Disposal Techniques

Proper containment and disposal of contaminated materials further reduce the risk of environmental or personnel exposure to oncological agents. The use of thick, plastic, sealable bags for initial containment of all waste is an easy and inexpensive way to enclose open ampuls, vials, and leaking IV tubing, bags and/or bottles. These bags can then be placed into larger, closed receptacles for disposal. Final disposal of oncological agents, as of all chemical hazards, is a subject of current controversy. The use of hazardous-waste incinerators that burn at extraordinarily high temperature seems to be the preferred method of disposal. Availability and expense of these units is a problem, however. The Environmental Protection Agency (EPA) allows the use of Class I, hazardous waste dump sites for toxic chemical waste but there are many readily apparent problems with burying any hazardous waste. Waste contaminated with oncological agents should not be treated as infectious waste since the methods of decontaminating infectious waste are ineffective with chemical hazards.

Information Is the Key

The success of any safety program depends on the understanding and
compliance of the workers. Orientation and training programs are of
primary importance in minimizing the occupational dangers of
handling oncological agents. Presentation of risks should be clear
and frank. Safety and emergency procedures should be thoroughly
explained and demonstrated. Compliance of workers to all aspects of
the program must be monitored.

CONCLUSIONS

Scientific evidence defining the dangers of continuous, low-level
occupational exposure to oncological agents is not yet available.
Research on occupational risks is difficult and continued exposure
of workers to a potential hazard, even for research purposes, could
impose a further legal liability on employers. For these reasons,
definitive studies of occupational exposure to oncological agents
may never be achieved.

Recommended safety precautions are neither prohibitively expensive
nor unreasonable. The health care industry should take the lead in
protecting workers from exposure to less than well-defined dangers
with the understanding that the quality of working life is not
always measured in dollars and cents.

REFERENCES

1. Denton DR. Are we killing the healers? Occup Health Saf.
    1982; 50:11-16 (Dec).

2. Harris CC. A delayed complication of cancer therapy - cancer.
    JNCI. 1979; 63(2): 275-7. Editorial

3. Falck K, Grohn P, Sorsa M et al. Mutagenicity in urine of
    nurses handling cytostatic drugs. Lancet 1979; i: 1250-51.

4. Crudi CB. A compounding dilemma: I've kept the drug sterile but
    have I contaminated myself? NITA. 1980; 3:77-78.

5. Ladik CF, Stoehr GP, Maurer MA. Precautionary measures in the
    preparation of antineoplastics. Am J Hosp Pharm. 1980;
    37:1184-86.

6. Kleinberg ML, Quinn MJ. Airborne drug levels in a laminar flow
    hood. Am J Hosp Pharm. 1981; 38:1301-3.

7. Neal A deW, Wadden RA, Chiou WL. Exposure of hospital workers
    to airborne antineoplastic agents. Am J Hosp Pharm. 1983;
    40:597-601.

8. Norppa H, Sorsa M, Vainio H, et al. Increased sister chromatid exchange frequencies in lymphocytes of nurses handling cytostatic drugs. Scand J Work Environ Health. 1980; 6(4):299-301.

9. Wasvik H, Klepp O, Brogger A. Chromosome analyses of nurses handling cytostatic agents. Cancer Treat Rep. 1981; 65:607-610.

10. Anderson RW, Puckett WH, Dana WJ, Nguyen TV, Theiss JC, Matney TS. Risk of handling injectable antineoplastic agents. Am J Hosp Pharm 1982; 39:1881-1887, 1982.

11. Staiano N, Galelli JF, Adamson RH. Lack of mutagenic activity in urine from hospital pharmacists admixing anti-tumor drugs. Lancet. 1981; i:615-6.

12. Sotaniemi EA, Sutinen S, Arranto AJ, et al. Liver damage in nurses handling cytostatic agents. Acta Med Scand. 1983; 214:181-9.

13. Hirst M, Tse S, Mills DG, et al. Occupational exposure to cyclophosphamide. Lancet. 1984; i:186-8.

14. Venitt S, Crofton-Sleigh C, Hunt J, Speechley V, Briggs K. Monitoring exposure of nursing and pharmacy personnel to cytotoxic drugs: urinary mutation assays and urinary platinum as markers of absorption. Lancet. 1984; i:74-77.

15. Editorial. How real is the hazard? Lancet 1984; i: 203.

16. Power LA, Stolar MH. Handling mutagenic drugs. Lancet. 1984; i: 560-70. Letter.

17. Brink CJ. Employee complaints draw OSHA inspections of hospital procedures for handling cytotoxic drugs. Am J Hosp Pharm. 1984; 41:591-2, 595, 608.

18. Power LA. Regulated handling of parenteral antineoplastic agents. Particulate and Microbial Control: Hospitals. 1983; 2:78-82.

19. Simonowitz J. Guidelines for preparation and administration of antineoplastic drugs. Cal/OSHA Medical Hazard Alert. June 17, 1983.

20. American Society of Hospital Pharmacists. Procedures for handling cytotoxic drugs. Bethesda, MD: American Society of Hospital Pharmacists; 1983.

21. ASHP technical assistance bulletin on handling cytotoxic drugs in hospitals. Am J Hosp Pharm. 1985; 42:131-7.

8

Asbestos Contamination of Drinking Water

JOSEPH LADOU

The carcinogenic hazards of asbestos exposure were first thought to apply to those inhaling the fibers in their work of from release of fibers in commonly used building materials. The hazards were slow to be recognized because the resultant carcinogenesis took many years to appear--for example, shipyard workers in World War II who were exposed to asbestos began to develop lung and gastrointestinal cancers only twenty or more years after exposure. More recently, the question arose as to whether or not the general population also was at risk because of the ingestion of asbestos in drinking water. This question was triggered by the finding from electron microscopic studies in 1973 that Lake Superior, which served as the municipal water supply to Duluth, Minnesota, and five small communities along the lakeshore, contained large amounts of amphibole asbestos fibers (Cook et al., 1974). The finding resulted in a series of studies covering a number of areas in North America that were suspected of having asbestos-contaminated water supplies.

Asbestos fibers enter the potable water system through geologic erosion of serpentine rock, environmental pollution (e.g., logging, mining, and dam-building), and erosion of asbestos-concrete pipes by corrosive water. Asbestos fibers are of two types: (1) chrysotile, or serpentine, asbestos with strong, flexible fibers that can be spun, and (2) amphibole asbestos derived from various silicates of magnesium, iron, calcium, and sodium, which generally are more brittle fibers that cannot be spun and are more resistant to chemicals and heat.

Available data on the concentration of asbestos fibers in U.S. drinking water supplies suggest that most water consumers are exposed to asbestos concentrations

of less than 1 million fibers per Liter. But a few
populations may be exposed to concentrations of more than
1 billion fibers/L, and some small water supplies in
northern California have asbestos concentrations of more
than 100 billion fibers/L (Millette et al., 1983). Of
the 538 water supplies for which asbestos contamination
data are available, 8 percent have fiber concentrations
higher than 10 million fibers/L.

The concern of the Environmental Protection Agency
and others is that the very long-term ingestion of asbestos-
contaminated water may result in gastrointestinal
carcinomas. The source of this concern is the high
incidence of these cancers in individuals who inhale
the fibers for long periods during their work, the
presumption being that fibers ejected from the lungs are
then swallowed. Both animal and epidemiologic studies
have been conducted to determine the long-term effects
of asbestos ingestion, but the findings to date have been
inconclusive.

Rats were most commonly used in the animal studies.
They ingested asbestos fibers in food or water for varying
lengths of time. Most of these studies indicated that
ingestion of the fibers failed to produce organ-specific
neoplasms. Their findings were either negative or
questionable. The problem may have stemmed from a number
of factors: (1) the use of differing strains of rats and
too small a number of experimental animals; (2) differences
in dose levels and asbestos fibers used; and (3) too short
a period of exposure (Condie, 1983).

Epidemiologic studies were made in Duluth, Minnesota;
the state of Connecticut; the San Francisco Bay Area; and
the Puget Sound Area, all of which have asbestos-contaminated drinking water.

In Duluth, the contamination of Lake Superior, the
drinking water source, occurred because of the dumping of
iron ore tailings begun in 1955 (Masson et al., 1974).
Asbestos in the drinking water amounted to about 8×10^6
TEM fibers/L. Cancer rates were studied for Duluth over
four 5-year periods covering the years between 1950 and
1969 (Masson et al., 1974). The data were separated by
body site of the cancer and by sex, and were compared
with cancer rates for the state of Minnesota and the
county of Hennepin where Minneapolis is located. But the
cancer mortality rates for Duluth did not differ significantly from those of the comparison areas, except for
cancer of the rectum, which the investigators concluded
was a "chance effect." A later study (Levy et al., 1976)
compared the rate of gastrointestinal cancer incidence in
Duluth to that of Minneapolis and St. Paul for the 1969 to
1971 period. Again, no consistent or significant
differences were observed, and the study added little to

the findings of Masson and co-workers.

Connecticut was studied for the incidence of gastro intestinal cancers in the population because of the use of asbestos-concrete pipe for delivering drinking water (Harrington et al., 1978). The study covered the years 1935 to 1973 and took into account such factors as the length and age of the pipes, and the ability of water to leach asbestos from the pipes. The study was limited by a lack of data on the actual amounts of asbestos in the water, with a generalization of ". . . below detectable limits (10,000 fibers per liter) to 700,000 fibers per liter." The relative risk of gastrointestinal cancers derived from asbestos in drinking water in this case has been estimated at 1.0006 (Safe Drinking Water Committee, 1983).

In the San Francisco Bay Area, drinking water is contaminated in certain parts of the area by the breakdown of naturally occurring serpentine rock. Some areas have shown asbestos contamination as high as 180×10^6 fibers/L (Kanarek et al., 1980). Statistics were obtained for the 722 census tracts of the San Francisco-Oakland Standard Metropolitan Statistical Area (SMSA). Observed or expected incidence of cancer were compared with measured asbestos counts in tract drinking water for the period 1969-1971. The study was flawed by the ever-increasing mobility of the population--that is, if 60 years is taken as the extreme of cancer exposure through ingestion, few of the population remained in the same census tract for anywhere near that length of time. Nonetheless, using this length of exposure, it has been estimated that the risk factors are 1.00, 1.00, 1.02, and 1.06 for the four levels of asbestos contamination in this area. Although observed ratios were about four times higher than the estimated risk factors, the ratios were modified by adjustments made for risk-modifying factors, such as mobility of the population. It would appear, therefore, that the estimated risk factors may be closer to reality, although still somewhat high. One finding of this study showed that lung cancer in males correlated strongly with asbestos-contaminated water even after adjusting for risk-modifying factors (Kanarek et al., 1980). The problem was attributed to the migration of ingested asbestos fibers to the lungs. However, the findings may also indicated that adjustments for some risk-modifying factors may not have been adequate. This conclusion appears to be supported by the study observation that cancer of the endometrium is negatively associated with the asbestos content of drinking water.

The Puget Sound Area is contaminated naturally by chrysotile asbestos (Polissar et al., 1982). The Sultan River flowing into the Sound is the primary source of contamination, with asbestos concentrations of 206×10^6 TEM fibers/L (samples obtained from tap water). The study compared cancer incidence statistics over the 1974-1977 period and cancer mortality from 1955-1975. Data were obtained from census tracts that received their drinking water from the Sultan River and compared them with census tracts in the Puget Sound Area where asbestos contamination of drinking water was much lower (7 x 10^6 TEM fibers/L). No significant findings of a correlation between asbestos-contaminated drinking water and the incidence of gastro intestinal cancer were found.

Thus, like the animal studies, the epidemiologic studies have been negative or equivocal in their findings. There may be a number of reasons for this failure in the human studies. The first is the dietary intake of asbestos fibers, which may be more common than realized. Food has several sources of asbestos contamination. In processed or filtered foods, the filtration process may be respon sible. Other sources are the cement floors, ceiling tiles, and pipe coverings. Foods that have been reported to contain asbestos fibers include vegetable oil, lard, mayonnaise, ketchup, talc-coated rice, and meat (Rowe, 1983). Beverages also may be contaminated including beer, some wines, and soft drinks (Wehman and Plantholt, 1979). Finally, asbestos fibers occur in oral medications containing talc (Eisenberg, 1974). Despite these findings and the suggestion that many, if not most, foods may be contaminated, few investigators have taken dietary intake of asbestos into account.

This may be only one of many reasons for the incon sistencies seen in the various studies. The resulting variations in interpretation of these studies have led to an understandable lack of regulatory concern. The National Research Council has suggested that the risk rate for gastrointestinal cancers from the daily consumption of 2 liters of water containing 0.11 x 10^6 TEM fibers/L over 70 years may result in one additional gastrointestinal cancer per 100,000 men or women (Safe Drinking Water Committee, 1983). The deficiencies of previous epidemio-logic studies must be avoided before it can be safely concluded that the ingestion of asbestos fibers in drinking water does not pose a significant cancer risk.

REFERENCES

1. Cook PM, Class JH, Tucker JH: Asbestiform amphibole minerals: Detection and measurement of high concen-trations in municipal water supplies. Science 185: 853-855, 1974.

2. Condie LW: Review of published studies of orally administered asbestos. Environmental Health Perspectives 53:3-9, 1983.

3. Eisenberg WV: Inorganic particle content of foods
    and drugs. Environmental Health Perspectives 9:183-
    191, 1974.

4. Harrington JM, Craun GF, Meigs JW: An investigation
    of the use of asbestos cement pipe for public water
    supply and the incidence of gastrointestinal cancer
    in Connecticut. Am J Epidemiol 107:96-103, 1978.

5. Kanarek MS, Comforti PM, Jackson LA, Cooper RS, Murchio
    JC: Asbestos in drinking water and cancer incidence
    in the San Francisco Bay Area. Am J Epidemiol 112:
    54-72, 1980.

6. Levy, BS, Sigurdson E, Mandel J, Laudon E, Pearson J:
    Investigating possible effects of asbestos in city
    water: Surveillance of gastrointestinal cancer
    incidence in Duluth, Minnesota. Am J Epidemiol 103:
    362-368, 1976.

7. Masson TJ, McKay FW, Miller RW: Asbestos-like fibers
    in Duluth water supply: Relation to cancer mortality.
    J Am Med Assoc 228:1019-1020, 1974.

8. Millette JR, Clark PJ, Strober J, Rosenthal M: Asbestos
    in water supplies of the United States. Environmental
    Health Perspectives 53:45-48, 1983.

9. Polissar L, Severson RK, Boastman ES, Thomas DB:
    Cancer incidence in relation to asbestos in drinking
    water in the Puget Sound Region. Am J Epidemiol 116:
    314-328, 1982.

10. Rowe JN: Relative source contributions of diet and
    air to ingested asbestos exposure. Environmental
    Health Perspectives 53:115-120, 1983.

11. Safe Drinking Water Committee, National Research
    Council: Epidemiology of the adverse health effects
    of arsenic and asbestos in drinking water. In:
    Drinking Water and Health, Vol. 5. Washington, D.C.:
    National Academy Press, 1983.

12. Wehman HJ, Plantholt BA: Asbestos fibrils in beverages.
    I Gin Bull Environ Contam Toxicol 11:267-272, 1974.

9

Environmental Agents in the Cause of Hepatic Malignancies

THOMAS D. BOYER

INTRODUCTION

In the following discussion I will review the role of environmental agents in the development of hepatocellular carcinoma (HCC). I will pay particular attention to the hepatitis B virus (HBV) as we have the clearest understanding of the relationship between HBV infection and HCC. Following a review of the epidemiologic evidence that supports the association of HBV and various environmental agents with HCC, the mechanisms of chemical carcinogenesis will be discussed briefly.

HEPATITIS B VIRUS

Viral Structure and Risk of Infection

The hepatitis B virus is a DNA virus that causes so called serum hepatitis in man. The virus is composed of an outer coat (hepatitis B surface antigen-HBsAg) and an inner core (hepatitis B core antigen-HBcAg). In addition, there is the hepatitis B e antigen (HBeAg) and a viral specific DNA polymerase. The circular partially double-stranded DNA is located within the core of the virus. In patients infected with the hepatitis B virus antibodies against the above antigens can be identified (1).

Following infection with HBV about 90% of the patients will have a self-limited illness with resolution of the hepatitis and clearing of the HBV. The remaining 10% will remain HBsAg positive for greater than 6 months (2). About half of this latter group of patients will eventually resolve the HBV infection. The remaining 5% will be chronic carriers for life and are at risk for the development of chronic liver disease and HCC.

HBV can be acquired by either percutaneous or nonpercutaneous means.
Percutaneous transmission is the most common and the various modes
of transmission include: blood products, intravenous drug use, hemodialysis, tattooing, acupuncture and insect bites. Nonpercutaneous
transmission occurs by the transfer of infected body secretions,
most frequently during intimate sexual contact.

Health care workers are at increased risk for being infected with HBV.
The risk is determined both by the length and type of practice. For
example, about 4-5% of physicians or dentists are anti-HBs positive
at the age of 30 whereas this rises to about 20% by the age of 50-
60 (3). The frequency of anti-HBs is 28% in surgeons, 18% in intern-
ists and only 4% in those involved in nonpatient care (Table 1) (4).
The highest incidence of anti-HBs positivity is in those who have
frequent contact with blood or blood products (5).

TABLE 1. Frequency of Hepatitis B Surface Antibody by Medical
Specialty

	Percent Positive
Surgery	28
Pathology	27
Pediatrics	21
Internal Medicine	18
Anesthesiology	17
Obstetrics	16
Family Practice	16
Nonpatient Care	4

From Denes et al. (4) with permission.

Association of HBV Infection and HCC

Infection with HBV is a world wide problem. In North, Central and
South America and Europe the prevalence of infection with HBV is low
(< 2%) whereas in South East Asia and Sub-Saharan Africa the incidence of infection with HBV is > 10% of the population (6). The
incidence of HCC parallels the infection rate of HBV with the annual
incidence in North America and Europe being relatively low, whereas
in South East Asia and Sub-Saharan Africa the incidence of HCC is
increased 10-20 fold.

The frequency of finding markers of HBV infection in the serum of
patients with HCC is high. In some studies, as many as 98% of the
patients with HCC will have some evidence of current (HBsAg) or past
(anti-HBc or anti-HBs) infection with the hepatitis B virus (6-8).
Also, family clustering of HCC and HBsAg positive carriers has been
reported (9,10). The mother is usually HBsAg positive (Table 2)
suggesting that in the patients developing HCC, infection occurred
by vertical transmission, probably during infancy (7).

TABLE 2.   HBsAg in Parents of HCC Patients and Carriers

	Mothers		Fathers		P Value
	HBsAg(+)/total	(%)	HBsAg(+)/total	(%)	
HCC	12/14	(86)	2/11	(18)	0.003
Carriers	17/49	(35)	9/42	(21)	0.244
P value	0.002		1.00		

Adapted from Beasley (7) with permission.

A number of investigators have looked for HBV antigens in the tumorous and nontumorous liver tissue of patients with HCC. HBsAg and less frequently HBcAg can be identified in the nontumorous tissue whereas the carcinoma cells infrequently contain HBsAg and apparently rarely HBcAg (11). Most recently integration of the HBV genome in both tumor and nontumorous cells has been demonstrated (12). The integration of HBV DNA has been demonstrated in patients with HBsAg in their serum whereas most patients with anti-HBs and HCC do not have integrated HBV DNA (12). In addition to patients, integrated HBV DNA has also been demonstrated in human hepatoma cell lines (13).

RNA tumor viruses (retroviruses) cause cancer in animals. They transform cells either because they contain an oncogene or by inte- gration of a viral promoter sequence next to a cellular proto- oncogene. There is no evidence that the HBV genome contains an oncogene. Although promoter sequences are present in the HBV genome, no sequences homologous to cellular proto-oncogenes have been shown to be adjacent to the integrated HBV sequence (12). DNA viruses transformation of infected cells is dependent upon the production of virus-coded transformation antigens. No transformation-like anti- gens have been produced in HBV infected cells (12). Hence, the role of integration in the transformation of hepatocytes to tumor cells remains poorly understood.

There are three viruses that are structurally similar to HBV and cause hepatitis in Pekin ducks (14), woodchucks (15), and ground squirrels (16). These viruses are called hepadna (hepatitis asso- ciated DNA) viruses. In the woodchucks, integration of the viral genome occurs and the animals also frequently develop HCC. However, in contrast to humans where tumors usually develop in cirrhotic livers, in the woodchuck there is no cirrhosis only acute and chronic hepatitis(12).

The strongest evidence that supports the role of infection with HBV in the pathogenesis of HCC is that of Dr. Beasley and colleagues (17). In 1975, a study was initiated in Taiwan. Male government employees were selected for a prospective study of the influence of HBsAg positivity on the subsequent development of HCC. 22,707 men were enrolled and tested for markers of infection with HBV. The participants were checked annually and cause of death determined from a review of hospital records. 3,454 of the participants were HBsAg positive and 113 of them developed HCC within 5 years of

entrance into the study. In contrast, of the 22,707 HBsAg negative
patients only 3 developed HCC in the same time period (Table 3).
The incidence was 527.7/100,00 population in the HBsAg positive
patients and only 2.6/100,000 in the HBsAg negative group. If the
variable of cirrhosis was added then the incidence in the HBsAg
positive patients increased to 2,419 per 100,000/yr (Table 3).

TABLE 3. HCC Incidence in Taiwan in Relation HBV Status and
Cirrhosis

Status	Number at Risk	HCC Number	Relative Risk	Incidence 100,000/yr
HBsAg+				
Cirrhosis	40	6	961	2,419
No Cirrhosis	3,414	107	201	505
HBsAg-				
Cirrhosis	30	0	-	0
No Cirrhosis	19,223	3	-	3

Adapted from Beasley and Hwang (17) with permission.

The data from Taiwan provides compelling evidence that infection
with HBV is associated with the subsequent development of HCC.
Infection with HBV however may not be the only factor in determining
whether HCC develops in a given patient. For example, HCC is less
common and occurs at an older age in urban population as compared to
a rural population. Kew et al (8) recently reported a study comparing rural to urban South African blacks with HCC. The peak incidence of the development of HCC was 20-50 years old ($\bar{x}=34.7$) in the
rural blacks, whereas it was 40-60 ($\bar{x}=50.9$) in the urban blacks.
The differences in age of onset could not be accounted for by the
differences in infection rates with HBV, and hence, the possibility
of a co-carcinogen, i.e., aflatoxin, was raised. The role of aflatoxin in causing HCC is discussed later in this chapter.

Hepatitis B vaccine. The HBV vaccine is derived from human carriers
of HBsAg. The HBsAg is separated from the complete virions by
isopyknic and rate zonal centrifugation. Following purification
the vaccine is inactivated by treatment with pepsin, 8 M urea and
formalin. Three doses of the vaccine are given and over 90% of the
recipients develop protective antibodies. The vaccine has been
shown to be safe and effective in preventing infection with HBV
(18). In the near future new HBV vaccines using recombinant DNA
technology should be available (19). The new vaccines will have
the advantage of not being derived from a human source and should
be less expensive and hence more likely to be used in Third World
countries where infection with HBV is a major public health problem.

CHEMICAL CARCINOGENS

Models

Chemically induced HCC in animals has been a popular experimental
model for the investigation of the developmental steps from normal
to malignant cells. Carcinogenesis is the end result of a number of
steps during which normal cells develop increasing degrees of auto-
nomy. The first step, called initiation, is assumed to lead to an
irreversible alteration in the cellular genome. These altered cells
usually are morphologically normal but are phenotypically changed.
They may express new proteins, such as α-glutamyltranspeptidase (20).
In addition, they develop certain characteristics that improves
their chances of survival compared to normal cells. The initiating
agent is a cellular toxin in addition to a carcinogen. After exposure to this injurious agent, the altered cells develop a consistent
change in the enzymes responsible for metabolizing hepatotoxins.
Most toxins require activation by so called phase I enzymes. In the
initiated cells, the levels of phase I enzymes are reduced by 80-90%.
The phase II enzymes which detoxify these noxious agents are, in
contrast, increased 2-6 fold compared to normal cells (21). Thus,
the pre-neoplastic cells have become resistant to toxic injury.

The initiated clones of cells will slowly disappear unless some other
event (promotion) follows initiation. The second event may stimulate
growth (phenobarbital, partial hepatectomy) or may select out clones
of resistant hepatocytes (CCl_4) (21). Interestingly, simple choline
deficiency may be the only stimulus required for initiated cells to
become malignant (22). It is important to note that all of these
events occur over prolonged periods of time with several weeks to
months required before HCC develops.

Human Carcinogens

Table 4 contains a partial list of agents that are known to cause
liver cancer in animals. Only four of the agents (arsenic, vinyl
chloride, thorotrast and aflatoxins) are well established human
hepatic carcinogens. Two of the agents, thorotrast (thorium
dioxide) and arsenic are largely assoicated with the development of
angiosarcomas and will not be discussed further.

Vinyl chloride. Vinyl chloride is a halogenated aliphatic hydrocarbon that causes both hepatic injury and liver cancer. At high
levels of exposure, vinyl chloride is oxidized by a P450 monooxygenase to a reactive species - chlorethylene oxide. This
reactive species may bind to proteins causing cell injury or to DNA
which presumably leads to the eventual development of cancer (23).

As with other carcinogens, vinyl chloride may also cause cell injury.
Acute exposure may cause mild elevations of serum transaminases
whereas with chronic injury, elevation of serum alkaline phospha-
tase and reduced hepatic clearance of indocyanine green are the

most common abnormalities. Animals and humans exposed to vinyl
chloride have developed HCC. However, angiosarcomas are much more
common and cofactors, such as ethanol, may be necessary for the
development of HCC (23).

TABLE 4. Environmental Agents and Liver Cancer

Hepatocellular Carcinoma		
Chemical Agents	Animal	Humans
Mycotoxins		
aflatoxin	+	+
sterigmatocystins	+	±
cyclochlorotine	+	±
Plant derived		
pyrrolizidine alkaloids	+	±
cycasin	+	±
Other compounds		
nitrosamines	+	±
acetylaminofluorene	+	±
polychlorinated bypheyls	+	±
vinyl chloride	+	±
Angiosarcomas		
Thorotrast		+
Arsenic		+
Vinyl chloride		+

List compiled from reference 24.

Aflatoxins. Aflatoxins are a family of mycotoxins produced by the
fungus Aspergillus flavus. The fugi grow on foodstuffs and the
resultant contamination leads to hepatic injury in man and animals.
As is true of most carcinogens, aflatoxins are hepatotoxins and it
was this latter characteristic that initially lead to their
discovery (24). Later it was discovered that the development of
liver tumors in hatchery raised trout was due to contamination of
their food by aflatoxins (24).

Aflatoxin B_1 (AFB_1) is the most potent member of this family. The
putative carcinogen is thought to be the 8,9-epoxide metabolite of
AFB_1. This metabolite then interacts with macromolecules, including
DNA. AFB_1 has been shown to bind covalently to DNA in vitro (25).
As with integrated HBV, however, it is unclear how this binding to
cellular DNA leads to cell transformation and eventually cancer.

The epidemiologic evidence is strong that a high intake of aflatoxin
is associated with an increase in the incidence of HCC. Contamination of foodstuffs with aflatoxin is uncommon in the Western
Countries, however, in the Far East many foods contain high levels
of aflatoxin (Table 5). In a case controlled study from the Philippines (26) the authors found that patients with HCC had a 4 fold
higher daily intake of aflatoxin compared to controls. A high

compared to a low consumption of aflatoxin appears to increase the
risk of developing HCC about 4-17 fold (24,26). The difficulty with
most of the studies on aflatoxin exposure is that no attempt was made
to control for HBV infection. As these studies come from areas
where HBV infection is prevalent, it is unclear whether aflatoxin
exposure alone can cause HCC in humans or whether it acts as a co-
carcinogen, perhaps by suppressing the immune response to HBV (27).
Alternately, exposure to aflatoxin is known to alter viral expression
in infected cells (28) and this may influence the subsequent development of HCC.

TABLE 5. Aflatoxin Content of Food in Philippines

	Meat Content (ppb)	% Positive
Cassava	467.5	100
Peanut butter	143.6	99
Yam	88.8	39
Sweet potato	60.6	84
Peanuts	49.1	70
Coffee, instant	11.2	53
Alcoholic drinks	1.9	47
Meat products	1.0	20

Adapted from Bulatao-Jayme et al (26) with permission.

Other associations between environmental agents and HCC. Recent
publications suggest that other agents not previously defined as
hepatic carcinogens may be associated with an increased risk of HCC.
Ethanol abuse is known to increase the risk of developing HCC. As
chronic alcoholism is associated with the development of cirrhosis
it is difficult to decide if the ethanol itself is a direct carcinogen (29). Ethanol abuse is also associated with the development
of cancer of the mouth, pharynx, esophagus and larynx. However,
smoking also is a significant factor in the development of the above
cancers and ethanol may be acting as a co-carcinogen. Similarly,
ethanol may also increase the risk of developing HCC in those with a
high intake of aflatoxin (26). Ethanol is known to induce the P450
monoxygenases and this might increase the rate of conversion of
aflatoxin to its toxic metabolite.

Recently, smoking has also been suggested to increase the incidence
of hepatocellular carcinoma (30,31). A study from the U.S. found a
2.6 fold increase in the risk of developing HCC in non-orientals who
smoked more than a pack of cigarettes each day. Ethanol abuse (> 80
g/day) increased the relative risk 4.2 fold and combined smoking
(> 1 pack/day) plus ethanol (> 80 g/day) increased it 14 fold (31).
Although HBsAg was not tested for in the latter study, in an earlier
study from Greece, smoking increased the risk of HCC about 5.5-fold
in patients who were negative for HBsAg (30).

I find it difficult to evaluate the true importance of smoking and
ethanol abuse in the pathogenesis of HCC, as ethanol and cigarettes

have not been shown to be or contain hepatic carcinogens. The above epidemiologic data does suggest, however, that other as yet undefined environmental agents may contribute to the development of HCC. The results of epidemiologic studies should stimulate more basic types of research to charcterize these new putative carcinogens.

CONCLUSION

Since the discovery by Blumberg in 1965, of the Australia antigen (HBV) the role of this virus in the pathogenesis of HCC has been extensively investigated. The presence of this virus in the liver has been shown to increase greatly the risk of developing HCC. In countries, such as Taiwan, where a large percentage of the population are infected with HBV, it is estimated that the lifetime risk of death either from HCC and/or cirrhosis is 40-50% for the male carriers (7). With the development of an effective vaccine, it becomes possible to reduce the world wide incidence of HCC by 80-90%. Reduced contamination of foodstuffs by aflatoxin should also reduce the incidence of HCC in certain areas of the world. Further reductions in the incidence of HCC await studies that define other environmental agents that cause HCC in humans.

REFERENCES

1.   Robinson, WS: Biology of human hepatitis viruses. In: Hepatology: A Textbook of Liver Disease, edited by D Zakim, TD Boyer, pp. 863-910. Philadelphia: Saunders, 1982.

2.   Redeker, AG: Viral hepatitis: clinical aspects. Am J Med Sci 270:9-11, 1975.

3.   Smith JL, Maynard JE, Berquist KR, Doto IL, Webster HM, Sheller MJ: Comparative risk of hepatitis B among physicians and dentists. J Inf Dis 133:705-706, 1976.

4.   Denes AE, Smith JL, Maynard JE, Doto IL, Berquist KR, Finkel AJ: Hepatitis B Infection in Physicians: Results of a nationwide seroepidemiologic survey. JAMA 239:210-212, 1978.

5.   Dienstag JL, Ryan DM: Occupational exposure to hepatitis B virus in hospital personnel: infection or immunization? Am J Epidemiol 115:26-39, 1982.

6.   Szmuness W: Hepatocellular carcinoma and the hepatitis B virus: evidence for a causal association. Prog Med Virol 24:40-69, 1978.

7.   Beasley RP: Hepatitis B virus as the etiologic agent in hepatocellular carcinoma-epidemiologic considerations. Hepatology 2:21S-26S, 1982.

8.   Kew MC, Rossouw E, Hodkinson J, Paterson A, Dusheiko GM, Whitcutt JM: Hepatitis B virus status of Southern African

blacks with hepatocellular carcinoma: comparison between rural and urban patients. Hepatology 3:65-68, 1983.

9. Denison EK, Peters RL, Reynolds TB: Familial hepatoma with hepatitis-associated antigen. Ann Intern Med 74:391-394, 1971.

10. Bancroft WH, Warkel RL, Talbert AA, Russell PK: Family with hepatitis-associated antigen. JAMA 217:1817-1820, 1971.

11. Popper H, Gerber M, Thung SN: The relation of hepatocellular carcinoma to infection with hepatitis B and related viruses in man and animals. Hepatology 2:1S-9S, 1982.

12. Sherman M, Shafritz, DA: Hepatitis B virus and hepatocellular carcinoma: molecular biology and mechanistic considerations. Semin Liver Dis 4:98-112, 1984.

13. Koshy R, Freytag von Lovinghoven ABL, Koch S, Marquardt O, Hofschneider PH: Structure and function of integrated HBV in genes in the human hepatoma cell line PLC/PRF/5. In: Viral Hepatitis and Liver Disease, edited by GN Vyas, JL Dienstag, JH Hoofnagle, pp. 265-276. Orlando: Grune and Stratton, 1984.

14. Mason WS, Seal G, Summers J: Virus of Pekin ducks with structural and biological relatedness to human hepatitis B virus. J Virol 36:829-936, 1980.

15. Summers J, Smolec JM, Snyder R: A virus similar to human hepatitis and hepatoma in woodchucks. Proc Natl Acad Sci USA 75:4533-4537, 1978.

16. Marion PL, Oshiro LS, Regnery DC, Scullard GH, Robinson WS: A virus in Beechey ground squirrels that is related to hepatitis B virus of humans. Proc Natl Acad Sci USA 77:2941-2945, 1980.

17. Beasley RP, Hwang L-Y: Hepatocellular carcinoma and hepatitis B virus. Semin Liver Dis 4:113-121, 1984.

18. Stevens CE, Taylor PE, Tong MJ, Pearl, TT, Vyas GN: Hepatitis B vaccine: an overview. In: Viral Hepatitis and Liver Disease, edited by GN Vyas, JL Dienstag, JH Hoofnagle, pp. 275-287. Orlando: Grune and Stratton, 1984.

19. Hilleman MR, Buynak EB, Markus HZ, Maigetter RZ, McAleer WJ, McLean AA, Miller WJ, Wampler DE, Weibel RE: Control of hepatitis B virus infection: vaccines produced from Alexander cell line and from recombinant yeast cell cultures. In: Viral Hepatitis and Liver Disease, edited by GN Vyas, JL Dienstag, JH Hoofnagle, pp. 307-314. Orlando: Grune and Stratton, 1984.

20. Goldfarb S: Biologic mechanisms of hepatocarcinogenesis. Semin Liver Dis 4:89-97, 1984.

21. Farber E: The biochemistry of preneoplastic liver: a common metabolic pattern in hepatocyte nodules. Can J Biochem Cell

Biol 62:486-494, 1984.

22. Takahashi S, Lombardi B, Shinozuka H: Progression of carci-
    nogen-induced foci of ∝-glutamyltranspeptidase-positive hepato-
    cytes to hepatoma in rats fed a choline-deficient diet. Int J
    Cancer 29:445-450, 1982.

23. Tamburro CH: Relationship of vinyl monomers and liver cancers:
    angiosarcoma and hepatocellular carcinoma. Semin Liver Dis
    4:158-169, 1984.

24. Newberne PM: Chemical carcinogenesis: mycotoxins and other
    chemicals to which humans are exposed. Semin Liver Dis 4:122-
    135, 1984.

25. Misra R, Muench KF, Humayun MZ: Covalent and noncovalent
    interactions of aflatoxin with defined deoxyribonucleic acid
    sequences. Biochemistry 22:3351-3359, 1983.

26. Bulatao-Jayme J, Almero EM, Castro MCA, Jardeleza MTR,
    Salamat LA: A case-control dietary study of primary liver cancer
    risk from aflatoxin exposure. Int J Epidemiol 11:112-119, 1982.

27. Lutwick LI: Relation between aflatoxin, hepatitis B virus and
    hepatocellular carcinoma. Lancet 1:755-759, 1979.

28. Rascati R, McNeely M: Induction of retrovirus expression by
    aflatoxin B_1 and 2-acetylaminofluorene. Mutation Res 122:235-
    241, 1983.

29. Kew MC, Popper H. Relationship between hepatocellular carci-
    noma and cirrhosis. Semin Liv Dis 4:136-146, 1984.

30. Trichopoulos D, MacMahon B, Sparro SL, Merikas G: Smoking and
    hepatitis B-negative primary hepatocellular carcinoma. JNCI
    65:111-114, 1980.

31. Yu Mc, Mack T, Hanisch R, Peters RL, Henderson BE, Pike MC:
    Hepatitis, alcohol consumption, cigarette smoking, and hepato-
    cellular carcinoma in Los Angeles. Canc Res 43:6077-6079, 1983.

10

Should Dietary Changes Be Recommended to Workers at Risk of Occupational Cancer?

ALLAN H. SMITH and JOSEPH W. SULLIVAN

1. INTRODUCTION

While the extent to which occupational exposures have caused
cancer is debatable, no one would question the importance of
reducing such risks. The first priority is clearly to prevent
occupational exposures to carcinogens, or to reduce exposures to
levels which make the risk of cancer so small as to be acceptable.

However, the question addressed in this paper concerns whether or
not the most one can do is prevent or reduce future exposures.
Must the worker with past carcinogenic exposures await what is
going to happen, or can his cancer risks be reduced? Survival
with cancer may be increased by early detection, and so medical
screening clearly has a place. Yet it would be of much greater
value if the actual risks of getting cancer could be reduced, and
dietary changes offer the most promise.

It has been estimated that at least 30% of current cancer deaths
might be prevented by dietary change (1,2). Some dietary constituents are carcinogenic, (3) and others protective. Of the
dietary components considered protective, micronutrients (vitamins, minerals and other trace elements), have figured prom-
inently. Currently, five particularly promising micronutrients are
being actively investigated, these include; carotene, vitamin A
and its synthetic analogs, selenium, vitamin C and vitamin E. The
next section will briefly examine the strength of the
micronutrient-cancer association for each of these elements by
reviewing the pertinent animal and human data. Following that,
reasons will be given as to why carotene will be emphasized as a
priority for intervention. High risk population groups including
cigarette smokers, and in particular cigarette smokers who have
also been exposed to asbestos, are then identified as target populations for intervention. The need for clinical trials is examined, but conclusions are drawn in the final section concerning
current intervention approaches for persons at risk of occupational cancer.

2. MICRONUTRIENTS IN THE PREVENTION OF CANCER

2.1. Carotene

Carotenoids are yellow plant pigments found in heavy concentration
in specific green/yellow fruits and vegetables. Several of these
can be metabolized to the physiologically active form of vitamin
A, retinol. Interest in the carotenoids as potential cancer
preventive agents was stimulated relatively recently when Peto and
Doll noted in their review (4) that most of the questionaires
employed in dietary vitamin A/cancer studies weighted carotene
sources of vitamin A (fruits and vegetables) far more than animal
sources, thus suggesting that these investigations provide
stronger support for the effect of the carotenes than for vitamin
A itself.

Some of the best epidemiologic evidence supporting a carotene-
cancer link comes from several early prospective dietary studies.
Bjelke (5) reported a five year follow-up on a cohort of 8278
Norwegian men who had replied to dietary and smoking postal questionaires. After controlling for smoking and age he noted that men
with the lowest "vitamin A" (actually carotene) consumption had a
relative risk for lung cancer three times higher than those men in
the highest intake group. A subsequent report on this cohort six
years later confirmed the initial findings (6). The largest prospective dietary study comes from Japan where 265,118 residents
completed an extensive dietary questionaire during the 1965 census
and were followed for a decade (7). A significant negative association was found for daily consumption of carotene containing
vegetables and cancer of the lung, stomach and prostate.

Only one prospective dietary study has attempted to differentiate
between the effects of carotene and preformed vitamin A on cancer
incidence (8). A cohort of 2107 employees at Western Electric
were followed for 19 years and a strong inverse association
between carotene intake and lung cancer were observed. Those in
the lowest carotene quartile were seven times more likely to get
lung cancer than those in the highest quartile. No protective
effect was found for intake of vitamin A itself.

Numerous retrospective dietary case-control studies support the
hypothesis that high carotene consumption is a protective factor
for a number of cancer sites including: lung (9-12); colon and
rectum (13); breast (14); larynx (15); cervix (16); oral (14); and
bladder (17). While these studies vary in their design, outcome
of interest and questionnaire format, each uses carotene sources
as their major measure of vitamin A intake. Furthermore only one
case-control study found no association between carotene and
cancer (18). However, when one examines each of the ten carotene
sources noted in this study, seven of these are negatively associated with GI cancer (p<.005).

Two prospective serum carotene studies have failed to show any
significant difference between the serum carotene of those who

subsequently develop cancer and those who do not (19,20). Several
small retrospective serum studies have shown a consistent difference between cases and controls (21-23). Unfortunately the lack
of power and other methodologic problems make their conclusions
difficult to evaluate.

The number of animal studies examining carotene's role in carcinogenesis are relatively few and focus on its ability to prevent or
delay the onset of skin or gastrointestinal tumors after exposure
to ultraviolet light or known carcinogens (24-28).

Before considering vitamin A itself, one intervention study
involving both carotene and vitamin A is worth noting, even though
it was not a controlled clinical trial. A group of betel nut and
tobacco chewers were given vitamin A and carotene supplements, and
it was found that the proportion of micronucleated buccal mucosal
cells decreased after treatment (29). While it is not clear
whether the effective agent was vitamin A or carotene, or both,
such studies may provide increasingly important evidence as to the
effectiveness of dietary interventions.

2.2. Vitamin A

Vitamin A is a fat soluble vitamin essential for normal cellular
differentiation. Hundreds of in vitro and animal studies have led
to the suggestion that vitamin A plays a key role in: suppression
of malignant phenotypic expression, suppression of proliferation,
stimulation of humoral and cellular immunologic defenses and the
restoration of contact inhibition. These studies have been
reviewed elsewhere (30-32).

The epidemiologic evidence in support of a vitamin A - cancer link
can be divided into dietary vitamin A studies and serum retinol
studies. Most of the dietary studies, as noted above, may provide
stronger evidence for carotene's cancer-preventive activity than
vitamin A's (4,33).

The early prospective serum retinol studies (34-37) each observed
a reduction in cancer risk for those with high serum retinol levels. Two recent reports however, found no risk reduction for
breast cancer (19) nor all cancers combined (20).

Finally, there have been a number of successful clinical trials
using analogs of vitamin A, suggesting that the retinoids may not
only be important in cancer prevevention but also may have a role
in chemotherapy (38-40).

2.3. Selenium

Selenium is an essential trace element whose role in cancer
prevention is thought to be mediated through its activity in the
enzyme glutathione peroxidase; an enzyme which minimizes intracellular oxidative tissue damage (3,41). Selenium has been shown to

reduce the mutagenic activity of several carcinogens (42) and to protect against a number of tumor inducing agents in animals (43,44).

The wide variation of soil selenium concentration within the United States has facilitated several ecologic studies which have noted lower age-adjusted cancer mortality rates in high and medium selenium areas (45,46). Furthermore, numerous case control studies have observed lower selenium levels in cancer patients compared with controls (47,48). In one prospective attempt to observe selenium's anti-cancer activity (49) 111 patients in whom cancer developed during a five year follow-up were found to have significantly lower serum selenium levels than 210 age, race, sex and smoking matched controls.

2.4. Vitamin C

In their 1979 review Cameron and Pauling promoted a cancer preventive role for vitamin C suggesting its involvement in numerous host-defense systems including: maintenance of the intracellular matrix, tumor encapsulation, enhanced immune competence, antiviral activity and the prevention of nitrosamine formation (50). Unfortunately, conflicting animal data and weak epidemiologic data have, as yet, been unable to confirm significant anti-cancer activity.

Several animal studies have found little or no effect of high dose vitamin C on cancer incidence (51,52). Others have actually noted enhanced tumor growth with vitamin C supplementation (53,54), while still others have observed an inhibitory effect of vitamin C on certain cancers (55).

The human epidemiologic evidence in support of the vitamin C hypothesis consists of a few ecologic studies (56) and numerous conflicting dietary case-control studies (57) which, as a rule, do not quantify vitamin C intake well and do not control for other dietary factors (eg carotene). To date, no long term prospective dietary studies have been reported and of the chemo-therapeutic trials published thus far, most have been negative (58,59).

2.5. Vitamin E

Vitamin E is an important intracellular anti-oxidant that has been shown to reduce mutations in bacterial testing systems as well as inhibit tumor formation in a small number of animal studies (60-62). Very few epidemiolgic studies concerning vitamin E have been carried out, but one recent prospective report found no relation between serum vitamin E levels and cancer incidence (20). However, another prospective serum vitamin E study found that the risk of breast cancer in women with vitamin E levels in the lowest quantile was about five times higher than the risk for women in the highest quantile (19).

3. REASONS FOR EMPHASIZING CAROTENE DIETARY INTERVENTION

The evidence cited above suggests that simple dietary changes in
the micronutrient consumption may dramatically reduce the risk of
many human cancers. While further information is needed before
specific micro-nutrient cancer associations can be considered conclusive, a question which must be addressed is; should one wait
years for the result of definitive clinical trials (63) or can one
already make sound, safe recommendations for dietary changes? In
order to assess this question we propose a four point scheme by
which potential dietary recommendations can be critically
evaluated. Each recommended dietary change in micronutrient consumption should:

(1) have reproducible animal and human data suggesting an anticar-
cinogenic effect.

(2) be feasible (e.g. have several available, palatable dietary
sources) with simple compliance requirements.

(3) be safe, even at extremes; and

(4) ideally result in additional health benefits.

While the first two requirements are concerned with the specific
soundness and feasibility of a long term intervention, the last
two principally address ethical issues in making such important
dietary recommendations. These standards ensure that even if no
reduction in cancer risk resulted from the recommended dietary
change that the individuals would be at no greater health risk and
that indeed, would benefit from the change. The remainder of this
section will be devoted to applying this scheme to each of the
micronutrients discussed above in order to determine which, if
any, should be included in new dietary recommendations.

3.1. Vitamin A

Vitamin A and the synthetic retinoids, as noted in the first section, are strongly implicated in both epidemiologic and animal
studies as important cancer preventive as well as chemotherapeutic
agents. The importance of this relationship is reflected in the
numerous ongoing clinical trials involving the retinoids (63).
Yet while the evidence supporting anti-cancer activity is strongly
suggestive, increased consumption of dietary preformed vitamin A
or vitamin A supplements cannot be recommended for several reasons. (Note: Pro-vitamin A, or carotene, will be discussed later.)

First, with the exception of the severely malnourished, serum
retinol is not affected by dietary intake (49). In other words,
doubling or tripling dietary intake of vitamin A would not substantially change serum concentrations, and is therefore unlikely
to change tissue levels. Secondly, large doses of vitamin A and
synthetic retinoids can result in serious acute or chronic hyper-
vitaminosis A syndromes (64). These problems with toxicity are

most profound with children (65,66). In addition, specific
retinoids have been identified as potential teratogens (67,68).
Finally, since major dietary sources of preformed vitamin A are
primarily from animal products high in fat and cholesterol, an
increase in preformed dietary vitamin A might actually increase an
individual's risks for CHD, obesity, breast cancer etc.

3.2. Selenium

Unfortunately, one is unable to recommend increasing dietary
selenium at this point for several reasons. Since there is a wide
variation of selenium in soils, forages and grains across the
U.S., one's serum level is highly dependent upon geographic location, source of produce and grains as well as diet. In the absence
of a high soil selenium area the most reliable way to consistently
increase serum levels is to take selenium supplements. Vitamin and
mineral supplements have a number of inherent problems, including
compliance and cost, but selenium supplementation has its own
specific hazards. Selenium in high doses has been shown to have
toxic and teratogenic effects in both animals and humans (69).
Also there is little evidence to suggest that selenium supplementation would benefit the health of an individual in any additional
way than its possible cancer protection.

3.3. Vitamin C

The epidemiologic studies involving physiologic doses of vitamin C
have, to date, shown little if any evidence suggesting a negative
association with cancer and only a limited association (recurrent
bladder Ca) at pharmacologic doses (57). While vitamin C is
readily available in many dietary sources and is safe in high
doses, early claims of vitamin C's activity in the prevention of
viral illnesses (the common cold) have largely been discredited
and no other potential benefit of high vitamin C intake has been
confirmed. Therefore because of a weak epidemiologic link and no
known additional health benefits associated with high vitamin C
consumption, it would be premature to advise an increase in
dietary vitamin C for the purpose of cancer prevention.

3.4. Vitamin E

The initial epidemiologic and animal studies, suggesting that
vitamin E's anti-oxidant activity may be protective against
cancer, need to be continued and confirmed before anything more
than a speculative outlook is warranted. However, if these studies
are confirmed, increased dietary vitamin E can be recommended as
it fulfills all of the remaining requirements outlined above.
First, it is readily available in large quantities in vegetable
oils and margarine and in moderate quantities in whole grains. It
has been shown to be safe at doses of fifty to seventy five times
the RDA.   60 And finally, if individuals switch form
saturated fats (butter) to poly unsaturated fats (vegetable oils
and margarine) they will not only increase their vitamin E serum
levels but will also reduce their risk for coronary heart disease

and obesity. Similarly, switching from white bread to whole grain
bread increases vitamin E while increasing dietary fiber with its
numerous health benefits (see next section).

3.5. Carotene

The last and by far the most promising group of micronutrients to
be discussed are the carotenes.

Several factors make dietary recommendation of increased carotene
consumption feasible. First, as demonstrated in table 1, there is
a wide variety of readily available and palatable sources of carotene. Secondly, as many of these foods are already part of a regular diet one would not have to acquire a taste for new foods or
pay for carotene supplements, thus ensuring better compliance and
greater likelihood of developing the ultimate goal of long-term
dietary change.

The safety of carotene consumption at high doses has been noted by
the FAD/WHO Expert Committee on Food Additives, who have estimated
the acceptable daily intake of beta carotene for an adult to be
350 mg per day while the average adult regularly consumes only a
few milligrams per day (4). The characteristic sign of excess
carotene consumption in whites is a canary yellow or golden
discoloration of the skin known as carotenoderma. Normal skin
coloration returns with the resumption of a normal diet (66). No
other signs or symptoms of toxicity has been regularly noted to be
associated with carotenemia.   70 However, one
recent report (71) noted amenorrhea associated with carotenemia in
a series of ten vegetarian patients. The small number of patients
and numerous uncontrolled potential confounders such as (1) weight
(two subjects 10% underweight) (2) heavy exercise (one subject
was a dancer) (3) prolonged oral contraceptive use (one subject
used OC's for the 8 years prior to amenorrhea) and other hormonal
disorders (one woman had mild hirsutism) make the validity of this
report difficult to evaluate.

In recommending an increase in carotene consumption one is, in
essence, simply recommending that a grater proportion of the diet
consist of specific fruits and vegetables. Several health bonuses
would result from following such a regimen. If one eats more
fruits and vegetables one is likely to eat less fatty food. This
change may help to reduce the severity of the diseases associated
with high fat diets such as obesity, coronary heart disease,
breast cancer etc. Similarly, as one increases their consumption
of fruits and vegetables their fiber intake increases propor-
tionately. Burkitt and others have proposed that high fiber diets
reduce: constipation, hiatus hernia, appendicitis, diverticular
disease and hemorrhoids (72). High fiber diets have also been
noted to reduce the risk of colon cancer (73) ,help lower serum
cholesterol (74,75) and help maintain glucose control in diabetics
(76,77).

A diet containing high amounts of carotene for the purpose of
cancer prevention can be justifiably recommended as it fulfills
the requirements of sound scientific foundation , feasibility,
safety and additional health benefits. Yet many may feel uneasy
about advising dietary changes to the general public in the
absence of conclusive scientific evidence

In anticipation of this criticism we suggest a more conservative
approach. That is, to restrict the dietary recommendations, at
present, to those individuals at high risk of cancer. In this
group the benefits of this safe dietary intervention will far
outweigh any potential risks. Examples of such high risk groups
will be discussed in the following section.

4. PERSONS WITH GREATEST NEED FOR CANCER RISK REDUCTION

Tobacco smoking is the single cause with the gratest proportion of
cancer incidence and mortality attributable to it. Between 25 and
40% of all cancer deaths in the United States are due to smoking
(2). In terms of numbers of people, the greatest need for cancer
risk reduction is among smokers. Stopping smoking is clearly the
most effective method for risk reduction, particularly since
cigarette smoke seems to influence late as well as early stages of
carcinogenesis, as evident by reductions in lung cancer risk
within 5 years of stopping smoking (78). In addition, both ex and
active cigarette smokers should be advised of the potential benefits of dietary changes in cancer risk reduction.

Smoking asbestos workers constitute a group in the population with
even greater cancer risks. Lung cancer mortality among cigarette
smoking asbestos insulation workers is over 50 times that for
non-smoking non-asbestos workers, and even non-smoking insulators
have experienced lung cancer mortality rates 5 times higher than
non-smoking non-asbestos workers (79). Admittedly, exposure to
asbestos has reduced markedly in recent years from that experienced by these insulators in the 1940's and 1950's, but the long
latency of asbestos induced cancer means that cases are still
occurring among workers with exposures in this era or soon after.
As well as lung cancer, asbestos exposure is associated with risks
of both pleural and peritoneal mesothelioma, cancers of the buccal
cavity, pharynx, larynx, esophagus, stomach, colon, rectum, and
kidney, to the extent that cancer mortality from all causes for
male asbestos insulators has been found to be as high as twice
that for the general population.

The first line of attack again must be reduction in asbestos exposure, and smoking cessation assistance. However parallel to such
activities, people with such high risks of cancer should be
advised that dietary change with increased carotene intake may be
beneficial. It is noteworthy that, apart from mesothelioma, there
is evidence of variable extent that carotene or retinol is protective against all the sites of cancer associated with asbestos
exposure.

An important question concerning risk reduction by dietary methods
is whether or not current dietary changes can influence cancer
risk due to exposures experienced 10, 20 or 30 years ago. We are
not aware of any animal evidence addressing this question, while
retinol or other micronutrients may be altered after carcinod
after carcinogen exposure in some animal studies, the time gap is
usually small. It appears, however, that carotene may exert an
effect on the later stages of carcinogenesis which gives hope that
risk reduction can indeed be accomplished many years after exposure, although further evidence is needed on this point.

5. THE NEED FOR CLINICAL TRIALS

Questions concerning cancer risk reduction by micronutrient
dietary interventions in humans can only be answered by clinical
trials. A variety of such studies are underway, or planned,
including studies of asbestos exposed workers. One of the the
studies being planned is a multicenter trial of carotene supplementation among workers with past heavy exposure to asbestos, with
follow-up for cancer outcomes. It is very important that such
studies go ahead, since if successful, they may provide evidence
which could lead to fully validated advice concerning cancer risk
reduction which could have major impact on future cancer incidence
throughout the world.

However, such studies are not without their problems. It will
only be possible to detect considerable reductions in cancer risk
with sufficient statistical power, of the order of 15-30%. Since
approximately 20% of deaths are due to cancer, even a small risk
reduction of 5-10% would be of public health importance. Another
problem is that to avoid being too prolonged, which would involve
considerable expense and problems with maintaining high participa-
tion rates, all the clinical trials are looking for a late carcinogenesis stage effect. For example, a study with 6 years of
follow-up must look for an effect within 6 years prior to clinical
diagnosis, even though the latency from cancer initiation may be
in excess of 30 years for many cases. More than that, statistical
power calculations for a 6 year follow-up study would rely on
effects during at least the last 3-4 years of follow-up, so reli-
ance is placed on their being an effect within the 2 year period
before a cancer would be clinically diagnosed if it had not been
prevented by the intervention.

Two questions therefore arise. In the light of the animal and
human evidence to date, can we wait until the results of definitive trails before recommending an intervention to high risk persons which involves no significant side effects? And even when we
have the findings from the clinical trials, would negative studies
mean that we should not recommend the intervention with carotene
in view of the problems described facing inference from the clinical trials? Answers to these questions should take into account
the fact that any major dietary changes in the general population
will reduce the likelihood of clinical trials yielding a definitive answer, in view of increased carotene intake in the placebo

or control group. However, the evidence which already exists cannot be hidden, and our actions on a clinical or public health
level must be responsive to the best information available.

6. CONCLUSION

There is a considerable body of animal and human evidence that a
variety of micronutrients play a protective role against cancer.
Carotene is one for which there is a growing amount of evidence
from prospective studies that high levels of dietary intake protect against cancer of the lung and other sites. In addition, the
dietary changes involved in increasing carotene intake, including
predominantly orange and green vegetables, have other beneficial
effects, in particular due to increased dietary fiber, but also
reduction in fat intake concomitant with reduced calories from
non-vegetable sources. Persons at high risk of cancer should
therefore be advised that dietary changes may reduce their cancer
risk. An important target group is cigarette smokers with past
asbestos exposure, although reductions or cessation of both exposures should be the first line of attack. Clinical contact with
patients at known high risk for cancer should include giving
dietary advice recommending increased consumption of carotene.

Table 1: Food Sources of Carotene

```
------------------------------------
                           ug/100g serving

Carrots              12,000
Spinach               6,000
Sweet potatoes        4,000
Broccoli              2,500
Cantalope             2,000
Apricot               1,500
Pumpkin               1,500
Mangoes               1,200
Lettuce               1,000
Tomatoes                600
Peaches                 500
Brussel sprouts         400
Cabbage                 300
Oranges                  50
Yams                     12
------------------------------------
```

REFERENCES

1. Wynder, EL, Gori, GB. Contribution of the environment to
   cancer incidence : an epidemiologic exercise. JNCI
   1977;58:825-832.

2. Doll, R, Peto, R. In: The causes of cancer: quantitative estimates of avoidable risks of cancer in the United States today. Oxford: Oxford University Press, 1981:1197-1308.

3. Ames, BN. Dietary carcinogens and anticarcinogens. Science 1983;221:1256-1264.

4. Peto, R, Doll, R, Buckley, JD, Sporn, MB. Can dietary beta-carotene materially reduce human cancer rates?. Nature 1981;290:201-208.

5. Bjelke, E. Dietary vitamin A and human lung cancer. Int J Cancer 1975;15:561-565.

6. Kvale, G, Bjelke, E, Gart, JJ. Dietary habits and lung cancer risk. Int J Cancer 1983;31:397-405.

7. Hirayama, T. Diet and cancer. Nutrition and cancer 1979;1:67-81.

8. Shekelle, R, Lepper, M, Liu, S, Mazlia, C, Raynor, WJ, Rossof, AH. Dietary vitamin A and the risk of cancer in the Western Electric study. Lancet 1981;2 :1185-1189.

9. Mettlin, C, Graham, S, Swanson, M. Vitamin A and lung cancer. JNCI 1979;62:1435-1438.

10. MacLennan, R, DaCosta, J, Day, NE, Law, CH, Ng, YK, Shanmugaratnam, K. Risk factors for lung cancer in Singapore Chinese : a population with high female incidence rates. Int J Cancer 1977;20:854-860.

11. Hinds, MW, Kolonel, LN, Hankin, JH, Lee, J. Dietary vitamin A, carotene, vitamin C and the risk of lung cancer in Hawaii. Am J Epidemiol 1984;119:227-237.

12. Gregor, A, Lee, PN, Roe, FJC, Wilson, MJ, Melton, A. Comparision of dietary histories in lung cancer cases and controls with special reference to vitamin A. Nutrition and Cancer 1980;2:93-97.

13. Graham, S, Dayal, H, Swanson, M, Mittelman, A, Wilkinson, G. Diet in the epidemiology of cancer of the colon and rectum. J Natl Cancer Inst 1978;61:709-714.

14. Marshall, J, Graham, S, Mettlin, C, Shedd, D, Swanson, M. Diet in the epidemiology of oral cancer. Nutrition and Cancer 1982;3:145-149.

15. Graham, S, Mettlin, C, Marshall, J, Priore, R, Rzepka, T, Shedd, D. Dietary factors in the epidemiology of cancer of the larynx. Am J Epidemiol 1981;113:675-680.

16. Marshall, JR, Graham, S, Byers, T, Swanson, M, Brasure, J. Diet and smoking in the epidemiology of cancer of the cervix. JNCI 1983;70:847-851.

17. Mettlin, C, Graham, S. Dietary risk factors in human bladder cancer. Am J Epidemiol 1979;110:255-263.

18. Modan, B, Cuckle, H, Lubin, F. A note on the role of dietary retinol and carotene in human gastro-intestinal cancer. Int J Cancer 1981;28:421-424.

19. Wald, NJ, Boreham, J, Hayward, JL, Bulbrook, RD. Plasma retinol, B-carotene and vitamin E levels in relation to the future risk of breast cancer. Br J Cancer 1984;49:321-324.

20. Willett, WC, Polk, BF, Underwood, BA, Stampfer, MJ, Pressel, S, Rosner, B, Taylor, JO, Schneider, K, Hames, CG. Relation of serum vitamins A and E and carotenoids to the risk of cancer. N Eng J Med 1984;310:430-434.

21. Ibrahim, K, Jafarey, NA, Zuberi, SJ. Plasma vitamin A and carotene levels in squamous cell carcinoma of oral cavity and oro-pharynx. Clinical Oncology 1977;3:203-207.

22. Lopez-S, A, LeGardeur, BY, Johnson, WD. Vitamin A status and lung cancer. Am J Clin Nutr 1981;34:641.

23. Mahmoud, LAN, Robinson, WA. Vitamin A levels in human bladder cancer. Int J Cancer 1982;30:143-145.

24. Santamaria, L, Bianchi, A, Arnaboldi, A, Andreoni, L, Bermond, P. Dietary carotenoids block photocarcinogenic enhancement by benzo(a)pyrene and inhibit its carcinogenesis in the dark. Experimentia 1983;39:1043-1045.

25. Rettura, G, Duttagupta, C, Listowsky, P, Levenson, SM, Seifter, E. Dimethylbenz(a)anthracene (DMBA) induced tumors : prevention by supplemental B-carotene (BC). Fed Proc 1983;42:786.

26. Mathews-Roth, MM. Antitumor activity of B-carotene, canthaxanthin and phytoene. Oncology 1982;39:33-37.

27. Mathews-Roth, MM. Carotenoid pigment administration and delay in development of UV-B-induced skin tumors. Photochemistry and photobiology 1983;37:509-511.

28. Epstein, JH. Effects of B-carotene on ultraviolet induced cancer formation in the hairless mouse skin. Photochemistry and Photobiology 1977;25:211-213.

29. Stich, HF, Rosin, MP, Vallejera, MO. Reduction with vitamin A and Beta-carotene administration of proportion of micronucleated buccal mucosal cells in Asian betel nut and tobacco

chewers. Lancet 1984;1:1204-1206.

30. Hicks, RM. The scientific basis for regarding vitamin A and its analogues as anti-carcinogenic agents. Proc Nutr Soc 1983;42:83-93.

31. Ong, DE, Chytil, F. Vitamin A and cancer. Vitamins and Hormones 1983;40:105-144.

32. Sporn, MB, Roberts, AB. Role of retinoids in differentiation and carcinogenesis. Cancer Res 1983;43:3034-3040.

33. Kummet, T, Moon, TE, Meyskens, FL. Vitamin A: evidence for its preventive role in human cancer. Nutrition and Cancer 1983;5:96-106.

34. Kark, J. The relationship of serum vitamin A and serum cholesterol to the incidence of cancer in Evans County, Georgia. PhD Dissertation, University of North Carolina, Chapel Hill., 1977.

35. Kark, JD, Smith, AH, Switzer, BR, Hames, CG. Serum vitamin A (retinol) and cancer incidence in Evans county, Georgia. JNCI 1981;66:7-16.

36. Wald, N, Idle, M, Boreham, J. Low serum vitamin A and subsequent risk of cancer. Lancet 1980;2:813-815.

37. Stahelin, HB, Buess, E, Rosel, E, Widmer, LK, Brubacher, G. Vitamin A, cardiovascular risk factors and mortality. Lancet 1982;1:394-395.

38. Alfthan, O, Tarkkanen, J, Grohn, P, Heinomen, E, Pyrhonen, S, Saila, K. Tigason (Etretinate) in prevention of recurrence of superficial bladder tumors. Eur Urol 1983;9:6-9.

39. Gouveia, J, Mathe, G, Hercend, T, Gros, F, Lemaigre, G, Santelli, G, Homasson, JP, Gaillard, JP, Angebault, M, Bonniot, JP, Lededente, A, Marsac, J, Parrot, R, Pretet, S. Degree of bronchial metaplasia in heavy smokers and its regression after treatment with a retinoid. Lancet 1982;1:710-712.

40. Kessler, JF, Meyskens, FL, Levine, N, Lynch, PJ, Jones, SE. Treatment of cutaneous T-cell lymphoma (mycosis fungoides) with 13-CIS-retinoic acid. Lancet 1983;1:1345-1347.

41. Chow, CK. Nutritional influence on cellular antioxidant defense systems. Am J Clin Nutr 1979;32:1066-1081.

42. Jacobs, MM, Matney, TS, Griffin, AC. Inhibitory effects of selenium on the mutagenicity of 2-acetylaminofluorene (AAF) and AAF derivatives. Cancer Letters 1977;2:319-322.

43. Shamberger, RJ. Relationship of selenium to cancer. 1. Inhibitory effect of selenium on carcinogenesis. JNCI 1970;44:931-936.

44. Helzlsouer, KJ. Selenium and cancer prevention. Seminars in Oncology 1983;10:305-310.

45. Shamberger, RJ, Willis, CE. Selenium distribution and human cancer mortality. CRC Crit Rev Clin Lab Sci 1971;2:211-221.

46. Schrauzer, GN, White, DA, Schneider, CJ. Cancer mortality correlation studies- 3 : Statistical associations with dietary selenium intakes. Bioinorganic Cemistry 1977;7:23-34.

47. Shamberger, RJ, Rukovena, E, Longfield, AK, Tytko, SA, Deodhar, S, Willis, CE. Antioxidants and cancer. 1. Selenium in the blood of normals and cancer patients. J Natl Cancer Inst 1973;50:863-870.

48. Broghamer, WL, McConnell, KP, Blotchky, AL. Relationship between serum selenium levels and patients with carcinoma. Cancer 1976;37:1384-1388.

49. Willett, WC, Stampfer, MJ, Underwood, BA, Taylor, JO, Hennekens, CH. Vitamins A, E and carotene: effects of supplementation on their plasma levels. Am J Clin Nutr 1983;38:559-566.

50. Cameron, E, Pauling, L, Leibovitz, B. Ascorbic acid and cancer. Cancer Res 1979;39:663-681.

51. Abul-Hajj, YJ, Kelliher, M. Failure of ascorbic acid to inhibit growth of transplantable and dimethylbenzanthracene induced rat mammary tumors. Cancer Letters 1982;17:67-73.

52. Reddy, BS, Hirota, N, Katayama, S. Effect of dietary sodium ascorbate on 1,2-dimethyl hydrazine- or methylnitrosourea-induced colon carcinogenesis in rats. Carcinogenesis 1982;9:1097-1099.

53. Migliozzi, JA. Effect of ascorbic acid on tumor growth. Br J Cancer 1977;35:448-453.

54. Banic, S. Vitamin C acts as a cocarcinogen to methylcholanthrene in guinea pigs. Cancer Letters 1981;11:239-242.

55. Pipkin, GE, Schlegel, JU, Nishimura, R, Shultz, GN. Inhibitory effect of L-ascorbate on tumor formation in urinary bladders implanted with 3-hydroxyanthranilic acid. Proc Exp Biol Med 1969;131:522-524.

56. Dungal, N, Sigurjonsson, J. Gastric cancer and diet: A pilot study on dietary habits in two districts differing markedly in respect of mortality from gastric cancer. Br J Cancer

1967;21:270-276.

57. Bright-See, E. Vitamin C and cancer prevention. Semin Oncol 1983;10:294-298.

58. Creagan, ET, Moertel, CG, O'Fallon, JR, Schutt, AJ, O'Connell, MJ, Rubin, J, Frytak, S. Failure of high-dose vitamin C (ascorbic acid) therapy to benefit patients with advanced cancer. N Eng J Med 1979;301:687-690.

59. Moertel, C, Fleming, TR, Creagan, ET, Rubin, J, O'Connell, MJ, Ames, MM. High dose vitamin C versus placebo in the treatment of patients with advanced cancer who have had no prior chemotherapy. N Eng J Med 1985;312:137-141.

60. Bieri, JG, Corash, L, Hubbard, VS. Medical uses of vitamin E. N Engl J Med 1983;308:1063-1071.

61. Cook, MG, McNamara, P. Effect of dietary vitamin E on dimethylhydrazine-induced colonic tumors in mice. Cancer Res 1980;40:1329-1331.

62. Haber, SL, Wissler, RW. Effect of vitamin E on carcinogenicity of methylcholanthrene. Proc Soc Exp Biol Med 1962;111:774-775.

63. DeWys, WD, Greenwald, P. Clinical trials: A recent emphasis in the prevention program of the National Cancer Institute. Semin Oncol 1983;10:360-364.

64. Olson, JA. Adverse effects of large doses of vitamin A and retinoids. Semin Oncol 1983;10:290-293.

65. Lippe, B, Hansen, L, Mendoza, G. Chronic vitamin A intoxication. Am J Dis Child 1981;135:634-636.

66. Elias, PM, Williams, ML. Retinoids, cancer, and the skin. Arch Dermatol 1981;117:160-180.

67. Rosa, FW. Teratogenicity of isotretinoin. Lancet 1983;2:513.

68. Hall, JG. Vitamin A teratogenicity. N Engl J Med 1984;311:797-798.

69. Buell, DN. Potential hazards of selenium as a chemopreventive agent. Semin Oncol 1983;10:311-321.

70. Lascari, AD. Carotenemia. Clin Pediatr 1981;20:25-29.

71. Kemmann, E, Pasquale, SA, Skaf, R. Amenorrhea associated with carotenemia. JAMA 1983;249:926-929.

72. Burkitt, D. Fiber as protective against gastrointestinal diseases. Am J Gastroenterol 1984;79:249-252.

73. Wynder, EL, Reddy, BS. Dietary fat and fiber in colon cancer. Semin Oncol 1983;10:264-272.

74. Jenkins, DJA, Leeds, AR, Newton, C, Cummings, JH. Effect of pectin, guar gum, and wheat fiber on serum cholesterol. Lancet 1975;1:1116-1117.

75. Anderson, JW, Chen, WJL. Plant fiber. Carbohydrate and lipid metabolism. Am J Clin Nutr 1979;32:346-363.

76. Anderson, JW, Ward, K. High-carbohydrate, high-fiber diets for insulin-treated men with diabetes mellitus. Am J Clin Nutr 1979;32:2312-2321.

77. Mahalko, JR, Sandstead, HH, Johnson, LK, Inman, LF, Milne, DB, Warner, RC, Haunz, EA. Effect of consuming fiber from corn bran, soy hulls, or apple powder on glucose tolerance and plasma lipids in type II diabetes. Am J Clin Nutr 1984;39:25-34.

78. Doll, R, Peto, R. Mortality in relation to smoking: 20 years' observations on male British doctors. Br Med J 1976;2:1525-1536.

79. Hammond, EC, Selikoff, IJ, Seidman, H. Asbestos exposure, cigarette smoking and death rates. Ann NY Acad Sci 1979;330:473-490.

11

Sunlight and Occupational Skin Cancer

C. G. TOBY MATHIAS

INTRODUCTION

The role of solar radiation in the induction of
cutaneous neoplasms was first noted in 1894 by Unna,
who observed degenerative and neoplastic changes in
sun-exposed areas of the skin of sailors, and later
by Dubreuilh, who described similar changes in grape
pickers (1). Since then, a considerable amount of
clinical, epidemiological, and experimental evidence
has accumulated establishing ultraviolet (UV)
radiation as one of our most important and potent
environmental carcinogens. Perhaps as many as 10-20%
of the total labor force in the United States
(currently about 100 million) are required to
perform some (or all) of their daily work outdoors.
Despite the large numbers of individuals
occupationally exposed to sunlight, and the more
frequent occurrence of skin cancers in those who
have worked outdoors (1), virtually no effort has
been made to protect workers' skins adequately from
carcinogenic UV radiation, nor is there any existent
legal requirement to do so. This seems somewhat
paradoxical considering the efforts and expenditures
to reduce and regulate occupational exposures to
substances which are only suspected to be
potentially carcinogenic in humans on the basis of
animal or laboratory studies.

Although other factors may contribute to the
development of cutaneous carcinogenesis, this review
will focus only on the clinical, epidemiological,
and experimental evidence which implicates sunlight
exposure in the pathogenesis of squamous cell, basal
cell, and melanoma skin cancer. Simple preventive
measures which should reduce the risk of developing
skin cancer in outdoor workers will be discussed.

CLINICAL EVIDENCE

Squamous cell carcinoma (SCC) of the skin is a tumor
of the squamous cells of the epidermis. It occurs
most frequently on areas of the body which are
chronically exposed to sunlight, i.e. the head,
neck, dorsal hands, and dorsal forearms.
Within anatomical areas of chronic exposure, there
is a further clustering of SCC development on
regions which receive maximal UV radiation: the
cheeks, nose, forehead, lower lip, and tops of the ears.
SCC seldom arises spontaneously on normal appearing
skin. Affected skin sites usually show signs of
extensive actinic damage. These include thickened,
yellowish, furrowed skin (solar elastosis), abundant
cutaneous wrinkles, multiple dilated superficial
blood vessels (telangiectasiae), solar induced
lentigines (freckles), and multiple flat,
erythematous, scaling, actinic keratoses, which are
premalignant precursor lesions to the development of
SCC. Clothing styles and cosmetic trends undoubtedly
are important determinants of the anatomical skin
sites which will receive maximum amounts of sunlight
exposure. Hair styles covering the ears and the use
of lipstick probably shield against enough UV
exposure to account for a lower   observed incidence
of SCC in these anatomical sites in women compared
to men (2).

Basal cell carcinoma (BCC) is a tumor of the basal
cell layer of the epidermis. BCC demonstrates a
similar strong clinical predilection for development
in anatomical skin sites chronically exposed to
sunlight. Unlike SCC, however, up to one third of
BCCs may develop in areas which are not chronically
exposed. Furthermore, there is a tendency for BCC to
cluster in periorbital skin or the nasolabial folds,
which receive considerably less UV exposure than
other areas of the face. Similarly, sites of BCC
occurrence may fail to show any signs of significant
solar elastosis or only minimal evidence of chronic
actinic damage. Because of these clinical
discrepancies, other factors in addition to UV
exposure probably contribute to BCC development (3).

Overall, the clinical evidence linking the
development of malignant melanoma (MM) to UV
exposure is less convincing. The most common
cutaneous sites of occurrence for the two principal
clinical variants of MM, superficial spreading (SSM)
and nodular (NM) melanoma are the trunk in
men, and the lower legs and back in women.
Lentigo maligna melanoma (LMM), a less common third
clinical variant, tends to occur almost exclusively

on chronically UV exposed areas of the face and neck
in older individuals. The incidence of MM on the
head and neck is rising more slowly than on the
trunk and lower limbs. These clinical trends are
consistent with a hypothesis implicating an
etiological role of UV radiation in MM, possibly
influenced by personal and social habits modulating
UV exposure, e.g. hair and clothing styles, or
intermittent exposure to large doses of UV radiation
on vacations, etc. (4).

EPIDEMIOLOGIC EVIDENCE

The risk for development of SCC, BCC and MM clearly
increases in Caucasian populations as one moves
closer to the equator (1,5,6), again suggesting that
increasing amounts of chronic UV exposure play an
important etiological role in the development of
these skin cancers. When the actual amounts of UV
radiation reaching the earth's surface at different
geographic locations are determined, corrected for
differences due to altitude or atmospheric
conditions at similar latitudes, the association
between annual UV exposure and the development of
skin cancer is even stronger (1). Within any given
geographic population of Caucasians, the risk of
developing SCC or BCC can be related to individual
cumulative outdoor exposure which results from
occupational or lifestyle considerations (5).
However, the ratio of BCCs to SCCs decreases as one
moves closer to the equator, rather than remaining
constant (1). This bit of epidemiological evidence
suggests that UV radiation is not nearly as
important in the pathogenesis of BCC as it is with
SCC.

Host factors which influence an individual's
susceptibility to actinic damage, such as degree of
skin pigmentation, ability to tan, and racial
origin, are other important determinants of risk for
developing skin cancer. SCC, BCC and MM are
relatively rare developments in Blacks and
Orientals. SCC and BCC occur more commonly in
Caucasians who tend to sunburn easily, and less
commonly in those whose skins tan readily (5). A
similar trend has been reported for MM (4), although
the data is less convincing. Caucasians descended
from Celtic (Irish, English, Scottish) origins also
have a clearly higher risk for the development of
SCC and BCC (5). When these risk factors are
combined with age, relative risks for developing SCC
or BCC may be estimated (7). A Caucasian over the
age of 60, who is pale complexioned, sunburns

easily, and has over 30,000 cumulative lifetime
hours of sun exposure, has a relative risk of
developing SCC of 347, and a relative risk of
developing BCC of 14.8.

EXPERIMENTAL EVIDENCE

SCC may be easily produced in hairless rodents by
repeated exposures to UV radiation (8), offering
convincing evidence of the fundamental role of UV
exposure in the pathogenesis of SCC. The primary
carcinogenic wavelengths are in the 290-320 nm (UVB)
range of the UV spectrum. Although wavelengths in
the 320-400 nm wavelength spectrum (UVA) are not
normally carcinogenic, except in extraordinarily
high doses, concomitant exposure to UVA may augment
experimentally induced UVB carcinogenesis (1,5,8).
Environmental changes induced by heat, wind, or
excessive humidity may also augment UVB induced
carcinogenesis in the laboratory (8).

To date, neither BCC nor MM has not been
experimentally reproduced in any animal species
following repeated exposures to UV radiation alone.
Melanocytic tumors indistinguishable histologically
from MM have been produced in hairless mice
following UV exposure after benign dermal
melanocytic tumors had already been induced by
repeated topical application of dimethylbenzanthracene.

Chemical substances known to be potent experimental
cutaneous carcinogens, such as polycyclic aromatic
hydrocarbons and nitrosourea compounds, have an
additive carcinogenic effect when combined with UV
exposure. Furthermore, other chemical substances
which are not primarily carcinogenic (e.g. croton
oil) may promote the development of UV induced
carcinogenesis (8). Thus, experimental data suggest
that a complex series of interactions of UV
radiation with other environmental substances may
be operative, and should be considered in any risk
assessment of skin cancer in the workplace.

The mechanism by which UV radiation induces skin
cancer formation is still unknown, but likely
involves either of two mechanisms, or a combination
of both. UV radiation readily induces dimer
formation in the skin; subsequent inhibition of
normal DNA repair may increase the chances of
cellular carcinogenic mutation. UV radiation also
generally induces a suppression of cell mediated
immune mechanisms in irradiated skin, which are
normally operative. Since immune surveillance may be

an important mechanism in cancer inhibition,
cutaneous immune suppression may also contribute to
the development of skin cancer.

PREVENTION

The most important aspect of any preventive program
aimed at reducing the risk of developing skin cancer
in the workplace should be reduction or prevention
of exposure to UV radiation. Outdoor work generally
must be performed during daylight hours in order to
take advantage of natural lighting, and potential
exposure to UV radiation is an inevitable
consequence of such work. Hats and tightly knit
clothing may stop most UV radiation, but in
warm or hot climates, workers often cannot tolerate
excessive clothing.

The most practical and efficient approach to
reducing UV exposure should be the regular use of a
protective sunscreen. The ideal protective sunscreen
should block not only UVB radiation, but also UVA,
and should resist being washed off the skin surface
by sweating, an invariable accompaniment of outdoor
work in warm climates. The most widely used
sunscreens are products containing p-aminobenzoic
acid (PABA) or its esters, benzophenones,
cinnamates, salicylates, and anthranilates. Only
commercial products containing benzophenones and
anthranilates provide sufficient protection against
UVA. The relative degree of photoprotection
provided by commercial sunscreens is usually defined
in terms of the ability to protect against acute
effects of UV radiation (i.e. sunburn), and is
expressed in terms of a solar protection factor
(SPF). The SPF is the ratio of the time required for
UV radiation to produce erythema through a sunscreen
to the time required to produce the same degree of
erythema without the sunscreen. SPF values range
from 2 (minimal protection) to 15 or more (maximal
protection). The SPF values displayed on commercial
sunscreen containers have usually been determined
indoors with UV radiation from an artificial light
source, and are generally greater than the true SPF
for the same sunscreen product used outdoors (9).
None of 30 products tested outdoors in one study had
an SPF greater than 12 (10). The relative resistance
to wash off may vary greatly from one commercial
sunscreen to another, and is not readily discernible
from sunscreen labels.

The experimental induction of skin cancer in rodents
following UV radiation may be inhibited by
sunscreens which block enough UV energy to prevent

erythema (9). However, enzymatic changes similar to
those seen in premalignant actinic keratoses may
still develop in photoprotected skin from small
suberythrogenic amounts of UV radiation which still
manage to penetrate the sunscreen (11). This
suggests that ideal photoprotection with sunscreens
should be aimed at reducing as much UV exposure as
possible, not just enough to prevent sunburn.

Table I contains a partial list of commercially
available sunscreens, with the outdoor SPFs as
determined by field testing and the relative sweat
resistances. In general, the most desirable
commercial sunscreens in terms of long term cancer
prevention should be those which block UVA as
well as UVB, which have the highest outdoor SPF, and
which have the best sweat resistance. Depending on
the SPF value and the length of exposure to UV
radiation, sunscreens may need to be reapplied
during the workshift. Since protection against UV
radiation is only relative, consideration should be
given to reapplication of the sunscreen when the
exposure time approaches one half the SPF value.

TABLE 1.   Selected Sunscreens and their Efficacies

Type/Trade Name	Photo-protection	SPF (Outdoors)	Sweat Resistance
PABA			
PreSun	UVB	6-8	excellent
Pabanol	UVB	6-8	fair
PABA ESTERS			
Original Eclipse	UVB	4-6	fair
Black Out	UVB	6	good
Pabafilm	UVB	4-6	good
Sundown	UVB	4-6	good
Sea and Ski	UVB	4	fair
NON-PABA			
Uval	UVB,UVA	4	poor
Coppertone	UVB	2	poor
Piz Buin 8	UVB,UVA	10-12	excellent
Ti Screen	UVB,UVA	10-12	excellent
PABA ESTER/NON-PABA COMBINATIONS			
Total Eclipse 15	UVB,UVA	6-9	excellent
PreSun 15	UVB,UVA	15	excellent
Sundown 15	UVB,UVA	10-11	excellent
Supershade 15	UVB,UVA	6-9	excellent
Clinique 19	UVB,UVA	7-8	good

Adapted from ref. 10.

REFERENCES

1. Harber LC, Bickers DR: Photosensitivity Diseases. Philadelphia, WB Saunders, 1981.

2. Stoll LH: Squamous cell carcinoma. In: Dermatology in Internal Medicine, edited by TB Fitzpatrick, AZ Eisen, K Wolff, IM Freedberg, and KF Austen, pp. 362-377. New York, McGraw Hill, 1979.

3. Van Scott EJ: Basal cell carcinoma. In: Dermatology in Internal Medicine, edited by TB Fitzpatrick, AZ Eisen, K Wolff, IM Freedberg, and KF Austen, pp. 377-383. New York, McGraw Hill, 1979.

4. Lee JAH: Melanoma and exposure to sunlight. Epidemiol Rev 4:110-136, 1982.

5. Urbach F, Epstein JH, Forbes PD: Ultraviolet carcinogenesis: experimental, global, and genetic aspects. In: Sunlight and Man, edited by TB Fitzpatrick, MA Pathak, LC Harber, et al, pp 259-282. Tokyo, Tokyo Press, 1974.

6. Sober AJ, Mihm MC, Fitzpatrick TB, and Clark WH: Malignant melanoma of the skin, and benign neoplasms and hyperplasias of melanocytes in the skin. In: Dermatology in Internal Medicine, edited by TB Fitzpatrick, AZ Eisen, K Wolff, IM Freedberg, and KF Austen, pp. 629-654. New York, McGraw Hill, 1979.

7. Vitaliano PP, Urbach F: The relative importance of risk factors in nonmelanoma carcinoma. Arch Dermatol 116:454-456, 1980.

8. Epstein JH: Photocarcinogenesis, skin cancer, and aging. J Am Acad Dermatol 9:487-502, 1983.

9. Sunscreens. The Medical Letter 26:56-58, 1984.

10. Pathak MA: Sunscreens: topical and systemic approaches for protection of human skin against harmful effects of solar radiation. J Am Acad Dermatol 7:285-312, 1982.

11. Pearse AD, Marks R: Response of human skin to ultraviolet radiation: dissociation of erythema and metabolic changes following sunscreen protection. J Invest Dermatol 80:191-194, 1980.

12

Phenoxyherbicides and Other Pesticides in the Etiology of Cancer: Some Comments on Swedish Experiences

LENNART HARDELL and OLAV AXELSON

INTRODUCTION

Untoward side effects of chemical preparations have become an increasing concern during the past decades. Especially the widespread use of herbicides, both for chemical warfare and for agricultural welfare, has caused a longlasting debate. A number of epidemiologic studies have appeared, especially about occupational cancer in various exposed worker groups. For example, Swedish railroad workers with exposure to amitrol, phenoxy acids and other herbicides were rather early found to have an increased cancer rate (Axelson and Sundell 1974; Axelson et al 1980) and lung cancers have been reported in excess among pesticide workers in DDR (East Germany; Barthel 1976, 1981).

Swedish Studies on Exposure to Chlorophenols and Phenoxy Acid Herbicides.

Further concerns about the health effects from especially phenoxy acids and chlorophenols arose in 1977, when a survey of soft tissue sarcoma patients revealed that they had quite often been in contact with these preparations (Hardell 1977), which have a chlorinated benzene structure in common and are partly produced through the same process. This observation initiated a number of case-referent (case-control) studies regarding exposure to chlorophenols and phenoxy acids as a potential risk factor for soft tissue sarcomas (Hardell, Sandstrom 1979; Eriksson et al 1981) and malignant lymphomas (Hardell et al 1981). A summary presentation of the studies is given in Table 1, where also a case-referent study on nasal and nasopharyngeal cancers in relation to chlorophenol exposure is included (Hardell et al 1982).

This latter study might be considered against earlier reports on nasal cancers, especially adenocarcinomas, among wood workers in the furniture industry, but also among leather and textile workers (c.f. Lancet Editorial 1983).

Table 1. Overview of results from Swedish studies on
chlorophenol and phenoxy acid exposure.

Chemical exposure	Type of cancer and place	Relative risk, 95% conf.interval	Reference
Phenoxy acids alone Chlorophenols alone	Soft-tissue sarcoma Northern Sweden	5.3.(2.4.-11.5) 6.6 (2.4-18.4)	Hardell, Sandstrom (1979)
Phenoxy acids alone Chlorophenols alone	Soft-tissue sarcoma Southern Sweden	6.8 (2.6-17.3) 3.3 (1.3-8.1)	Eriksson et al 1981
Phenoxy acids alone Chlorophenols alone	Malignant lymphoma Northern Sweden	4.8 (2.9-8.1) 8.4 (4.2-16.9)	Hardell et al 1981
Phenoxy acids alone Chlorophenols alone	Nasal and naso- pharyngeal cancer Northern Sweden	2.1 (0.9-4.7) 6.7 (2.8-16.2)	Hardell et al 1982
Phenoxy acids alone Chlorophenols alone	Colon cancer Northern Sweden	1.3 (0.6-2.8) 1.8 (0.6-5.3)	Hardell 1981
Phenoxy acids alone Chlorophenols alone	Primary liver cancer Northern Sweden	1.7 (0.7-4.4) 2.2 (0.7-7.3)	Hardell et al (1984)

Cabinet making is a relatively uncommon occupation in northern
Sweden, where this study was conducted. In addition, few hard
woods have been used in the furniture industry in that part of the
country. However, the excess of nasal and nasophayngeal cancers
was found to be related to chlorophenol exposure as obtaining in
the saw-mills, where the control for bluestain and mould in newly
cut and sawn timber usually was based on chlorophenol treatment
until the end of 1977. Furthermore, high levels of chlorinated
dibenzodioxins and dibenzofurans, constituting impurities in
chlorophenols, have been found in the dust from saw mills in
Sweden (Levin et al 1976). In this context of nasal and
nasopharyngeal cancers it might be added that whole-body
autoradiography in mice has shown the
2,3,7,8-tetrachloro-dibenzo-p-dioxin (TCDD) to accumulate
particularly to in the nasal mucosa (Appelgren et al 1982). The
earlier found nasal cancer risk among cabinet makers refers
particularly to adenocarcinomas, whereas the epidermoid type of
cancer tended to predominate in our study. Hence, our findings
do not seem to be related to woodwork as such, but rather to work
in those saw mills using chlorophenols.

The referents of the nasal and nasopharyngeal cancer study were
the same as those utilized in the studies of soft-tissue sarcomas
and lymphomas in Northern Sweden, a circumstance that will be

somewhat further discussed with regard to validity aspects and in
relation to a contemporary undertaken study of colon cancer.

The Swedish studies of soft-tissue sarcomas and lymphomas have
created much discussion, and they have prompted close surveys of
similarly exposed populations in various parts of the world. As
a result, a few cases of soft-tissue sarcomas and also lymphomas
have been discovered in worker groups with exposure to
chlorophenols (Honchar and Halperin 1981). A cohort study of
persons employed in the manufacture of phenoxy herbicides in
Denmark showed also an excess of cases with soft-tissue sarcoma
(Lynge 1984). Case reports tend to be an uncertain basis for
conclusions on causality, however, and there is not yet any
published, definite support for the Swedish epidemiologic
observations. Recently a positive association between herbicide
exposure and ovarian mesotheliomas was reported in a
case-referent study (Donna et al 1984).

There are, however, a couple of non-positive studies, one of them
a cohort of phenoxy acid sprayers from Finland (Riihimaki et al
1982), the other a case-referent study on soft-tissue sarcomas
and phenoxy acid exposure from New Zealand (Smith et al 1984),
although "potential exposure" to chlorophenols as occurring in
tanneries and meat works pealt departments gave an odds ratio
of 7.2. in the New Zealand study. Nor did Milham (1982) find any
clear evidence for a relation between soft-tissue sarcomas,
chlorophenols and phenoxy acids in a proportional mortality
evaluation from Washington State, i.e. when just using
occupational titles as a crude exposure variable. a quite recent
communication from Gallagher and Threlfall (1984) suggests an
excess of lymphosarcomas and reticulosarcomas among sawmill
workers in British Columbia, Canada, although no excess of
soft-tissue sarcomas could be identified in their investigation.

It might be a remark of interest in this context that the high
rate ratios in the Swedish studies are reduced below 2, if just
the occupational titles of forestry and farming are used as the
exposure variable; c.f. Table 2. Hence, there is actually no
direct contradiction between the findings from Sweden and the
state of Washington.

Some Methodological Aspects

Risk evaluations, particularly about the use of phenoxy acid
herbicides, have been undertaken in many countries and have
consequently brought up various concerns about validity in the
Swedish studies. For example, Coggon and Acheson (1982), raised
the question of a possible observational bias, i.e. the
possibility of a misclassification of exposure either dependent
on a memory bias among the subjects interviewed and/or due to the
possibility that the investigators would have had a tendency,
conscious or not, to ascribe exposure to the cases more readily
than to the referents.

It is "well known" or at least a common belief, that case
referent studies should be particularly prone to false
results because of misclassification of exposure. It might
be noted then, that just a random misclassification would
result in a less sensitive study, i.e. the estimate of the
risk ratio would tend to be biased towards unity, although
it could happen just by chance, that also a rather high risk
estimate would be obtained.

The latter is hardly any explanation for the high risk ratios in
the Swedish studies, since it is extremely unlikely that the
whole series of studies should have a random misclassification in
the same direction and of considerable magnitude. Therefore it
merely remains to look for some sort of a systematical
misclassification, i.e. a tendency for cases to report exposure
and for referents to rather neglect or disregard experiences with
chlorophenols or phenoxy acids or, alternatively, the
investigators could have been prone to misclassify as discussed
above.

With regard to chlorophenol exposure in saw mills, there was an
opportunity to compare the exposure data obtained from
questionnaires with information from the employers but no
important differences were detected (Hardell, Sandstrom 1979).
For persons stating forest work questionnaires were sent to
employers in order to verify their employment and possible
exposure. Answers were obtained for only 4 of 10 cases and 16 of
40 referents (40%). Regarding exposure to phenoxy acids this
method gave a crude rate ratio of 21.0. Due to the low response
rate no conclusions could be drawn, however (c.f. Hardell,
Sandstrom 1979). In two of the studies (Eriksson et al 1981,
Hardell, et al 1981) also a special epidemiologic technique
(Axelson 1980; c.f. also Tockman 1982), was applied to check for
the possibility of an observational bias. The principle of this
technique is that if cases from among the occupations of forestry
and farming were apt to exaggerate their phenoxy acid exposure,
there would be a relative deficit of unexposed cases within these
worker groups and, conversely, there would be too many, falsely
unexposed referents within these occupations. Such a situation
would be reflected in a formal prevention for the
non-exposed in forestry and farming together with a falsely
elevated risk among the exposed, all in comparison to other,
potentially unexposed occupations. No such phenomena could
be identified in the studies with regard to phenoxy acid
exposure, but this technique was not so easily applicable
with regard to chlorophenols as used in variety of
occupations; c.f. Table 2.

Furthermore, it has been found that questionnaire data for
case-referent studies might be much more adequate than usually
thought, judging from a direct comparison of information obtained
from questionnaires with that of employee registers (Pershagen,
Axelson 1982).

Table 2. Exposure to phenoxy acids in cases and referents by
occupation in one of the soft-tissue sarcoma studies (Eriksson et
al 1981) and in the lymphoma study (Hardell et al 1981). Ph=
phenoxy acids, Ch= chlorophenols, unexp= unexposed

	Agric/forestry			Other Occupations		
	Ph	Ch	Unexp	Ph	Ch	Unexp
Soft tissue sarcomas	13	1	17	1	10	68
Referents	5	3	39	0	5	167
Risk ratio	6.4	–	1.1	–	4.9	(1.0)
Lymphomas	35	5	37	6	15	71
Referents	23	1	114	1	7	189
Risk ratio	4.1	–	0.9	–	5.7	(1.0)

NOTE: Considering occupations in agriculture and forestry only,
the risk ratios reduce to (31) (172)/(47)(79) = 1.4 for
soft-tissue sarcomas and to (77) (197)/(138)(92)=1.2 for the
lymphomas with regard to phenoxy acid exposure

Other steps were also taken to identify the possibility of
an observational bias in the soft-tissue sarcoma and
lymphoma studies, namely by applying the same questions and
epidemiological methods in reference to another cancer form,
i.e. colon cancer (Hardell 1981). At least the great
majority of colon cancer cases would conceivably not have
any relation to chlorophenols or phenoxy acid herbicides.
If individuals suffering from cancer would be generally apt
to over report exposure, an effect would have appeared also
with regard to this malignancy, but no such observation
could be made in spite of a contemporary, intensive debate
in the mass media on the adverse effects of these compounds,
c.f. Table 1. Moreover, the aforementioned study of nasal
and nasopharyngeal cancer was undertaken concommitantly with
the colon cancer study, i.e. the questionnaires were
simultaneously sent out to both these groups of cases and
any supplementary telephone interviews regarding exposure
for the two series of cancer cases were mixed and made by
the same interviewers in a blinded manner. Also a case-
referent study on primary liver cancer was non-positive regarding
an association with exposure to phenoxy acids or chlorophenols
(Hardell et al 1984).

In our soft-tissue sarcoma studies all cases were included
regardless of anatomical location. In the first study (Hardell,
Sandstrom 1979) 18 out of 52 cases (35%) and in the second study
(Eriksson et al 1981) 52 of 110 cases (47%) were coded on other
sites than ICD 171. Consequently, for example a number of cases

with leiomyosarcoma or neurogenic sarcoma were included in the
studies. Since only cases 26 years and older were included no
childhood sarcomas were involved. All the histopathological
specimens were reviewed thus verifying the diagnosis and allowing
for the most up-to-date classification of soft-tissue sarcomas.

Of interest is the distribution of exposure to phenoxy acids in
cases and referents over the years prior to diagnoses of the
respective case. In figure 1 latency periods in the first
soft-tissue sarcoma study (Hardell, Sandstrom 1979) are given
divided in 5 year groups. The maximum duration of latency was 27
years corresponding to the time when phenoxy herbicides were
introduced in Swedish forestry. Days of exposure to phenoxy
acids are given for cases and referents within each 5 year period
taking into account the matching number of 4 referents to each
case. Maximum exposure in cases was between 15-20 years prior to
the diagnosis. If exposure data were mainly due to recall bias
one should expect most of the exposure to be reported only a few
years prior to diagnosis since the concept of latency period in
chemical carcinogenesis is generally not known in the population.

Median latency periods for exposure to phenoxy acids and
chlorophenols are presented in Table 3. Further investigations
should thus allow for a latency period of approximately 20 years.
In a recent study by Greenwald et al (1984) on soft-tissue
sarcoma and exposure to Agent Orange in Vietnam the maximum
latency period was 13 years and mean only 10 years. That study
can thus not answer the question if exposure to Agent Orange is a
risk factor for soft tissue sarcoma. Some of the cases were even
diagnosed prior to most of the use of Agent Orange in Vietnam.

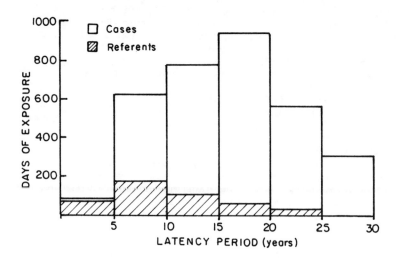

Figure 1. Latency periods for exposure to phenoxy acids in the
first soft-tissue sarcoma study (Hardell, Sandstrom 1979).

Table 3. Median latency periods (years) in Swedish studies; soft-tissue sarcoma (STS) I = (Hardell, Sandstrom 1979), STS II = (Eriksson et al 1981), malignant lymphoma = (Hardell et al 1981)

	STS I	STS II	Malignant lymphoma
Phenoxy acids	15	20	19
Chlorophenols	21	25	22

New information from Denmark and British Columbia (Olsen, Jensen 1984; Gallagher, Thelfall 1984) certainly provides some refutation to the Swedish findings about nasal and nasopharyngeal cancer but a crucial question is of course whether or not dioxins are present in the wood dust. This might not necessarily be the case, since there seems to be mainly hardwood dust exposure in the Danish furniture industry and in British Columbia, chlorophenol impregnation is used for protecting the timber from molds during transportation, i.e. impregnated timber should preferably not be further worked on before exportation. Furthermore, epidemoid cancers should be considered separately from the hardwood related adenocarcinomas, before any further conclusions can be reached in this context.

The Scientific Debate

With regard to the precautions taken to avoid observational bias, it is remarkable that quite critical but nevertheless superficial statements tend to appear from time to time in evaluations of these studies, e.g. "Because public awareness of the risks from 2,4,5-T herbicides have been acute for some years, there is a probability that a bias from exposure recall occurred in both studies" (Advisory Committee on Pesticides 1982). Even more unspecified criticism can be found like "These three studies have been criticized widely and have been accused of being subject to both observer and recall bias along with the possibility of selection bias" (The Herbicide Committee of the Iverness-Victorial Medical Society, Canada 1983). It is possible that some of these pseudoarguments may derive from a rather biased information provided in a well known scientific journal, but in an unsigned article, which had merely the character of an advertisement by a herbicide producer (Anonymous 1981), or by other critical view-points that have gone into the literature (Hay 1982). Still, it had been prudent and certainly to the benefit of epidemiology if various evaluations had been more specific and profound.

In the retrospect, it still seems rather unlikely that a traditional type of observer or recall bias should explain the results of these studies, nor is there any other convincing possibility for bias. Confounding from another risk factor is a possibility but is not likely to have

produced an effect of this magnitude. Nor is there any
reason to believe that a selectional bias should have
operated, although it has been proposed that cases of
soft-tissue sarcomas and lymphomas from the upper social
classes, not exposed to chlorophenols or to phenoxy acids, would
have had their treatment in other regions of Sweden. However,
the national health care system along with the compulsory
registration of cancers with regard to, among other things, the
domicile of the case does definitely exclude such a possibility
as an explanation for the findings. Nevertheless, there could
still remain some sort of an unrecognized, systematical error in
these studies, and, if so, its sound identification would be very
valuable both for the epidemiological methodology and for the
risk assessment with regard to chlorophenols and phenoxy acid
herbicides.

Chemical and Biochemical Considerations

Unless the findings of the relationships between lymphomas,
soft-tissue sarcomas, nasal and nasopharyngeal cancers and
exposure to chlorophenols and phenoxy acid herbicides (except for
the nasal and nasopharyngeal cancers in this latter respect)
finally turn out to be explicable through the recognition of some
bias in the epidemiological technique, there remains to identify
the specific etiological factor. Common to phenoxy acids and
chlorophenols has been a content of chlorinated dibenzo-p-dioxins
but one should perhaps not necessarily consider only the well
studied, most toxic 2,3,7,8-tetrachlorodibenzo-p-dioxin (TCDD) in
this context, but also other dioxins could be of interest, e.g.
2,7-dichlorodibenzo-p-dioxin and mixtures of
hexachlorodibenzo-p-dioxins, especially as indications also have
been obtained of a carcinogenecity from these derivatives (NIH
1979, NIH 1980). TCDD is now known to be an extremely potent
promoter and able to produce malignancies in mice and rats,
including sarcomas (Van Miller et al 1977; Kociba et al 1979; NIH
1982 a, b). This promoting capacity of TCDD is shared with some
of its approximate isostereomeres, which like TCDD effectively
induce microsomal monooxygenase activity (Poland et al 1979,
Poland et al 1982). Furthermore, there might be some sort of
interaction with vitamin A, since TCDD-effects also have some
similarities with vitamin A deficiency and vitamin A compounds
(retinoids) may inhibit cancer promoters. Deficiency states have
also been related to increased rates of lung and stomach cancer
(c.f. Thunberg 1983 for further details and references).

It is of further interest in this context that results are under
way from analyses of chlorinated dibenzodioxins and dibenzofurans
in abdominal fat both from cases of soft-tissue sarcoma and
malignant lymphoma and from a group of control patients suffering
from gallbladder diseases or cancer (Hardell et al 1985). Among
7 cases with soft-tissue sarcoma or malignant lymphoma exposed to
phenoxy acids 16 to 31 years ago the levels of
1,2,3,6,7,8-hexachlorodibenzodioxin (HxCDD) were significantly
higher than among the control patients unexposed to phenoxy
acids. Also the 2,3,4,7,8-pentachlorodibenzofuran (PeCDF) and

1,2,3,6,7,8-hexachlorodibenzofuran (HxCDF) were significantly
higher in the exposed cases versus the unexposed controls. No
differences in cases and controls were found for TCDD. In
general the levels of the higher chlorinated dioxin isomers were
higher than the lower chlorinated both in cases and controls
indicating some kind of environmental exposure to the population.
The most likely sources of the higher chlorinated dioxin isomers
are incineration, impurities from chlorinated phenols and PCBs
(c.f. Ryan et al 1985).

The levels of TCDD in our study did not correlate well with
previous exposure to phenoxy acids. The half life time of TCDD
in human adipose tissue is not known but based upon animal data
one should expect exposure to phenoxy acids long time ago not to
be reflected by increased levels of TCDD in adipose tissue (Piper
et al 1973 a,b). Of interest is, however, that dermal absorption
of TCDD in backpack sprayers could be of the same magnitude as
the level inducing tumors in animals (c.f. Backstrom 1980).

It is certainly also worth notice that nitrosamines have been
found in some phenoxy acid herbicide preparations in Sweden
(Osterdahl, Dich 1982), but if one would suggest the nitrosamines
to be responsible for the observed malignancies, no clear
connection would be obtained to the observations made for the
chlorophenols. There might also be a possibility that
combinations could be formed with other substances, capable of
causing cancer, since at least in plants, conjugations of phenoxy
acids with aminoacids are known to occur and there has been some
indication of similar reactions also in experimental animals
(c.f. Aberg, Eliasson 1978 as well as Rappe 1978).

Another explanation for the observed malignancies could have to
do with the stimulatory effect of phenoxy acids as well as of the
drug clofibrate on peroxisome proliferation. Hence clofibrate
like other hypolipidaemic, hepatic peroxisome proliferators is
known to be carcinogenic, presumably through producing hydrogen
peroxide, increasing the formation of reactive oxygene radicals
(Reddy and Azarnoff 1980; c.f. also Linnainmaa 1983). The
problem is again however, that there is no specific information
available in this respect with regard to the effect of
chlorophenols and in view of the epidemiologic findings, it seems
necessary to be able to find a cancer mechanism in common for
both types of preparations. As the facts stand today, it seems
as if the content of dibenzodioxins and/or furans in both the
phenoxy acids and the chlorophenols would constitute the best
explanation for the observed carcinogenic properties from these
preparations.

Epilogue

In Sweden, 2,4,5-T was withdrawn in early 1978, mainly on
political grounds, but also the chlorophenols were banned in the
beginning of 1978. The reason for both these decisions seems to
have been a general concern for the contents of dioxin impurities
along with the risk of getting such compounds synthesized by

burning wood treated with chlorophenols. There were also some
complaints about diffuse symptoms like irritation of the skin and
airways, headache and gastrointestinal complaints among saw mill
workers at the time, which seems to have further strengthened the
decision to cancel the registration of the chlorophenols. Hence,
there is now a decreasing opportunity for further studies in
Sweden on this matter as relating to occupational epidemiology,
but hopefully studies in other countries would provide final
understanding of the health hazards, especially the cancer risk,
that, by now at least, seems to be associated with the use of
these compounds.

REFERENCES

Aberg B, Eliasson L. The herbicidal effect of phenoxy compounds.
In: Ramel C (ed) Chlorinated phenoxy acids and their dioxins.
Ecological Bulletins 27: 86-100., 1978

Advisory Committee on Pesticides (Kilpatrick R). Report on
phenoxy acid herbicides. Ministry of Agriculture, Fisheries and
Food, London (unpublished report), 1982.

Anonymous Swedish studies discounted in 2,4,5-T risk
assessment..42: A-32., 1981.

Appelgren L E, Brandt I, Brittebo E B, Cillner M, Gustavsson J A.
Autoradiography of 2,3,7,8-tetrachloro (14C) dibenzo-p-dioxin
(TCDD): Accumulation in the nasal mucosa. 3rd International
Symposium on Chlorinated Dioxins and Related Compounds
(Abstracts). Salzburg Oct 1982.

Axelson O. A note on observational bias in case-referent studies
in occupational health epidemiology. Scand Work, Environ Hlth 6:
80-82, 1980.

Axelson O, Sundell L. Herbicide exposure, mortality and tumor
incidence: An epidemiological investigation on Swedish railroad
workers. Work, Environment, Health 11: 21-28., 1974

Axelson O, Sundell L, Andersson K, Edling C, Hogstedt C, Kling H.
Herbicide exposure and tumor mortality. An updated epidemiologic
investigation on Swedish railroad workers. Scand. J. Work
Environ Hlth 6: 73-79., 1980.

Backstrom J. Synpunkter rorande eventuella halsorisker vid
anvandning av fenoxlsyrapreparat. Swedish Industrial Chemical
Association 1980, not published (in Swedish)

Barthel E. Gehauftes Vorkommen von Bronchialkrebs bei
beruflicher Pestizidexposition in der Landwirtschaft.
Zeitschrift fur Erkrankungen der Atmungsorgane 146: 266-274.,
1976

Barthel E. Increased risk of lung cancer in pesticide exposed
male agricultural workers. Hlth 8: 1027-1040, 1981

Coggon D, Acheson E D. Do phenoxy herbicides cause cancer in man? Lancet i: 1057-1059., 1982

Donna A, Betta PG, Robutti F, Crosignani P, Berrino F, Bellingeri D. Ovarian mesotheliai tumors and herbicides: a case-control study. Carcinogenesis 5: 941-942, 1984

Eriksson M, Hardell L, Berg N O, Moller T, Axelson O. Soft tissue sarcomas and exposure to chemical substances; a case-referent study. Br. J. Ind. Med. 38: 27-33., 1981

Gallagher R P, Threlfall W J Cancer and occupational exposure to chlorophenols. Lancet ii: 48. 1984.

Greenwald P, Kovasznay B, Collins DN, Therriault G. Sarcomas of soft tissue after Vietnam service. JNCI 73: 1107-1109, 1984

Hardell L Malignant mesenclymal tumours and exposure to phenoxy acids. A clinical observation (in Swedish, English summary). Lakartidningen 74: 2753-2754, 1977

Hardell L Relation of soft-tissue sarcoma, malignant lymphoma and colon cancer to phenoxy acids, chlorophenols and other agents. Scand J. Work Environ Hlth 7: 119-130., 1981

Hardell L, Sandstrom A Case-control study: Soft tissue sarcomas and exposure to phenoxyacetic acids or chlorophenols. Br.J. Cancer 39: 711-717., 1979

Hardell L, Eriksson M, Lenner P, Lundgren E Malignant lymphoma and exposure to chemicals, especially organic solvents, chlorophenols and phenoxy acids: A case-control study. Br J. Cancer 43: 169-176., 1981.

Hardell L, Johansson B, Axelson O. Epidemiological study of nasal and nasopharyngeal cancer and their relation to phenoxy acid or chlorophenol exposure. Am. J. Ind Med 3: 247-257., 1982.

Hardell L, Bengtsson NO, Jonsson U, Eriksson S, Larsson LG. Aetiological aspects on primary liver cancer with special regard to alcohol, organic solvents and acute intermittent porphyria-an epidemiological investigation. Br J Cancer 50: 389--397, 1984.

Hardell L, Domellof L, Nygren M, Hansson M, Rappe C. Levels of polychlorinated dibenzodioxins and dibenzofurans in adipose tissue of patients with soft-tissue sarcoma or malignant lymphoma exposed to phenoxy acids and of unexposed controls. 1985. To be published.

Hay A. The chemical scythe. Lessons of 2,4,5-T and dioxin. p. 178, Plenum Press, New York and London. 1982

The Herbicide Committee of the Iverness-Victorial Medical Society. Health effects of herbicides 2,4-D and 2,4,5-T. Report to the Nova Scotia Forestry Commission, Canada (unpublished report), 1983

Honchar P A, Halperin W E 2,4,5-T, trichlorophenol and soft-tissue sarcomas. Lancet i: 268-269, 1981

Kociba R J, Keyes D G, Beyer J E, Carreon R M, Gehrin P J Long-term toxicologic studies of 2,3,8-tetrachloro-dibenzo-p-dioxin (TCDD) in laboratory animals. Annals of New York Academy of Sciences 320: 397-404, 1979.

Lancet editorial. Towards control of nasal cancer. Lancet i: 856-957, 1983.

Levin J O, Rappe C, Nilsson C A. Use of chlorophenols as fungicides in sawmills. Scand J Work Environ Hlth 2: 71-81, 1976

Linnaimaa K. Genotoxicity of phenoxy acid herbicides 2,4-D and MCPA. Dissertation; University of Helsinki and Institute of Occupational Health, Helsinki. 1983

Lynge E. Ukrudtsmidler og kraeft. The Danish Cancer Registry, Denmark 1984 (In Danish, English summary)

Milham S Jr. Herbicides, occupation and cancer. Lancet i: 1464-1465. 1982

NIH Bioassay of 2,7-dichlorodibenzo-p-dioxin for possible carcinogenecity. National Toxicology Program, Technical Report Series No. 123, 1979

NIH Bioassay of a mixture of 1,2,3,6,7,8 and 1,2,3,7,8,9-hexachlorodibenzo-p-dioxins for possible carcinogenecity (gavage study). National Toxicology Program, Technical Report Series No. 198, 1980

NIH Carcinogenesis bioassay of 2,3,7,8-tetrachloro-dibenzo-p-dioxin in Swiss-Webster mice (dermal study). National Toxicology Program, Technical Report Series No. 201. 1982a

NIH Carcinogenesis bioassay of 2,3,7,8-tetrachloro-dibenzo-p-dioxin in Osborne-Medel rats and B6C3F, mice (gavage study). National Toxicology Program, Technical Report Series No. 209. 1982b.

Olsen J H, Moller Jensen O. Nasal cancer and chlorophenols. Lancet ii: 47-48. 1984

Osterdahl B G, Dich J. Occurrence of nitrosamines in some pesticides. (In Swedish, English summary) Vaxtskyddsrapporter, Jordbruk 20: 185-188, 1982

Pershagen G, Axelson O. A validation of questionnaire information on occupational exposure and smoking. Scand J Work, Environ Hlth 8: 24-28, 1982

Piper, W.N., Rose, J.Q. & Gehring, P.J. Excretion and tissue distribution of 2,3,7,8-tetrachlorodibenzo-p-dioxin in the rat. Environm. Hlth Perspect., 5, 241-244, 1973a

Piper, W.N., Rose, J.Q. & Gehring, P.J. Excretion and tissue distribution of 2,3,7,8-tetrachlorodibenzo-p-dioxin in the rat. Advanc. Chem. Ser., 120, 85-91, 1973b

Poland A, Greenlee W F, Kende A S Studies on the mechanism of action of the chlorinated dibenzo-p-dioxins and related compounds. Annuals of New York Academy of Sciences 320: 214-230. 1979.

Poland A, Palen D, Glover E. Tumour promotion by TCDD in skin of HRS/J hairless mice. Nature 300: 271-273. 1982

Rappe C. Chemical background of the phenoxy acids and dioxins. In: Ramel C (ed): Chlorinated phenoxy acids and their dioxins. Ecological Bulletins 27: 28-30., 1978.

Reddy J K, Azarnoff D L. Hypolipidaemic hepatic peroxisome proliferators form a novel class of chemical carcinogens. Nature 283: 397-398., 1980.

Riihimaki V, Asp S, Hernberg S. Mortality of 2,4-dichlorophenoxyacetic acid and 2,4,5-trichlorophenoxyacetic acid herbicide applicators in Finland. First report of an ongoing prospective study. Scand J. Work, Environ Hlth 8: 37-42., 1982.

Ryan JJ, Lizotte R, Lau B P-Y. Chlorinated dibenzo-p-dioxins and chlorinated dibenzofurans in Canadian human adipose tissue. Chemosphere 1985, (In press).

Smith A H, Pearce N, Fisher D O, Giles H J, Teague C A. Soft-tissue sarcoma and exposure to phenoxyherbicides and chlorophenols in New Zealand. JNCI 73: 1111-1117, 1984

Thunberg T. Studies on the effect of 2,3,7,8-tetrachlorodibenzo-p-dioxin on vitamin A: A new aspect concerning the mechanism of toxicity. Dissertation; Karolinska Institute, Stockholm. 1983

Tockman M S. Epidemiology in the workplace: The problem of misclassification. J. Occup. Med. 24: 21-24., 1982

Van Miller J P, Lalich J J, Allen J R. Increased incidence of neoplasma in rat exposed to low levels of 2,3,7,8-tetrachlorodibenzo-p-dioxin. Chemosphere 10: 625-632., 1977.

13

Smoking and Occupational Lung Cancer

NEAL L. BENOWITZ

INTRODUCTION

One hundred years ago the first automatic cigarette rolling mach-
ines began operation. Mass production and marketing of cigarettes
ushered in a 100-year epidemic that has resulted in millions of
premature deaths world-wide. Because of the lag in the appearance
of smoking-related disease, it took more than 50 years before the
risks of cigarette smoking were clearly established (Hammond and
Horn, 1958). Even though some progress has been made in reducing
cigarette smoking since its peak in the 1950's (Harris, 1983), the
incidence of some smoking related diseases, such as lung cancer, is
still rising (American Cancer Society, 1983).

The importance of smoking as a contributor to occupational lung
disease has been recognized only in the past 15 years. That smoking
and occupation should be additive in causing disease is to be expected. If risks of smoking and occupation are additive, the worker
may argue that smoking is a personal choice so long as he is willing
to risk the health consequences. But several studies indicate a
synergistic or multiplicative effect of smoking and occupational
toxin exposures. Because certain cancers would not have occurred
without the combination of occupational exposure and cigarette smoking, these cancers must be considered occupation-related cancers.
Smoking is, therefore, a cause of occupational cancer. Since industry and workman's compensation are financially responsible for occu-
pationally-induced illnesses, smoking becomes a concern of the
employer.

Exposure of the nonsmoker to cigarette smoke is well known to be a
source of annoyance. Recent studies indicate that passive smoke
exposure may also result in impairment of pulmonary function and
possibly lung cancer in the nonsmoker. A workplace in which the
nonsmoker is exposed to cigarette smoke is, therefore, a hazardous
workplace. No longer is the right of the smoker to freedom of
choice in personal habits the overriding consideration.

A few industries have cigarette smoking control policies. Those who do, do so primarily to protect products or clients or to meet legislated workplace requirements. But workplace control of smoking could substantially reduce occupational work hazards, and smoking control policies make good economic sense.

SMOKING AND CANCER

It has been estimated that smoking is responsible for 30% of cancer in the United States today (Doll and Peto, 1981). As much as 80 or 90% of lung cancers, 75% of oral, laryngeal and esophageal cancers, and 50 to 60% of bladder and kidney cancers have been attributed to smoking (Table 1). Lung cancer incidence most clearly illustrates the smoking-cancer connection. Incidence of most types of cancers has been relatively constant in the United States since 1900, but the lung cancer rate has been steadily rising (American Cancer Society, 1983). The rise in lung cancer rate parallels the average per capita consumption of cigarettes, with a lag of 20-30 years (Figure 1). Smoking prevalence for men peaked in 1950-60, but because of a lag, lung cancer rate is still rising today. Women took up smoking later as a group than men and, as a result, lung cancer rates have more recently began to increase for women.

HOW DOES CIGARETTE SMOKING CAUSE CANCER?

Tobacco smoke and smoke condensate produce cancer in experimental animals (Hoffmann et al., 1978). The combustion of tobacco results in generation of over 3,000 chemicals. These are for the most part chemicals that are present in the environment whenever organic material is burned. The greatest contributors to the carcinogenesis of tobacco condensate appear to be the polyaromatic hydrocarbons, the most potent of which is benzo(a)pyrene (Hoffmann et al., 1978).

TABLE 1. Cancer Related to Smoking

Site	Relative risk	% Deaths Attributable
Lung	10	90
Laryngeal	20*	
Oral	6*	75
Esophageal	4*	
Bladder	3	56
Kidney	2	–
Pancreatic	2	40
Stomach	1.4	–
Uterine Cervix	2	–

*   Alcohol acts synergistically (Surgeon General, 1982).

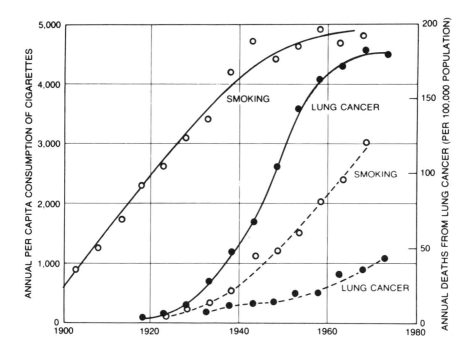

FIGURE 1. Temporal relationship between cigarette consumption and death rate from lung cancer. Solid lines represent men, dashed lines women. Data are for England and Wales (Cairns, 1975).

Tobacco smoke also contains catechols, metals (nickel, cadmium and arsenic), radiation sources (polonium 210) and a number of gases which are mutagenic or carcinogenic (Table 2). Nicotine may act as a cocarcinogen and nitrosated derivatives of the tobacco alkaloids, including N'-nitrosonornicotine and 4-(methylnitrosamino)-1-(3-pyridyl)-1-butanone, are potent carcinogens specific to tobacco.

Carcinogenesis is most likely when tumor initiators are delivered in high concentration to a target organ and in the presence of tumor promoters. Tobacco smoking is ideal for carcinogenesis. Carcinogens and cocarcinogens are effectively delivered to the airways via inhaled cigarette smoke. A number of tumor promoters are also supplied to permit completion of the carcinogenesis process. Nonspecific pulmonary effects, including chronic inflammation with generation of oxygen-free radicals and impaired pulmonary clearance of carcinogens may also contribute (Kilburn, 1984). Autopsy studies have indicated that dysplastic lesions occur at the site of chronic inflammation (Auerbach et al., 1979). These are thought to be premalignant, preceding the development of squamous cell carcinoma.

TABLE 2. Mutagens and Carcinogens in Tobacco Smoke

Particulate Phase	Vapor Phase
Polynuclear Aromatic Hydrocarbons*	Hydrazine*
Catechols	Formaldehyde*
Nicotine	Urethane*
N-Nitrosonornicotine	Vinyl Chloride*
Nickel (Carbonyl)*	Nitrosodiethylamine
Cadmium*	Aromatic Amines
Arsenic*	(2-Naphthylamine)*
Polonium-210*	Nitrogen Oxides*

*   Potential occupational and environmental exposures

Since inflammation may predispose to development of lung cancer, nitrogen oxides, acrolein and other irritants may also be important in carcinogenesis.

There may have been a change in histologic type of lung cancer in smokers over recent years, with greater occurrence of adenocarcinoma (Wynder and Goodman, 1983). This is also the type of cancer which occurs most commonly in people with passive cigarette smoke exposure. Adenocarcinomas are located more peripherally in the lung, suggesting that gaseous components rather than particulates may be etiologic.

Tobacco smoke carcinogens and occupational toxins may interact in several ways. As seen in Table 2, most of the potentially carcinogenic substances in tobacco smoke may be found in some workplace environments. This should result at a minimum in an additive risk of smoking and occupational exposures. If, as currently thought, carcinogenesis depends on exposure to both initiators and promoters, smoking may provide the cocarcinogen and/or tumor promoter which is needed to complement actions of occupational carcinogens. Tobacco smoke may also be the vehicle for transmission of occupational carcinogens into the lung. Finally, cigarette smokers may be more tolerant to noxious substances in the air, allowing greater exposure to environmental carcinogens.

SMOKING IN THE WORKPLACE

Currently in the United States about 30% of adults smoke cigarettes (Harris, 1983). The distribution of smokers in various occupations is not homogeneous. Persons who are better educated and have white collar jobs are less likely to smoke (Covey and Wynder, 1981; Sterling and Weinkam, 1976). For example, in a recent survey of practicing pulmonary physicians only 4.6% were cigarette smokers (Sachs, 1983). Blue collar workers (excluding farmers) are most likely to smoke, and their cigarettes are more likely to be high tar cigarettes. Rates of smoking in particular industries have been as high as 80% in some studies (Pastorino et al., 1984). In the United States today about 45% of blue collar workers smoke. Unfortunately, the latter group is the one most likely to be exposed to occupational chemical carcinogens.

SMOKING AND WORKPLACE CANCER

Interaction of smoking and occupational exposures in cancer causation has been examined for some occupational toxins. In several studies there is evidence suggesting multiplicative effects. In other studies, smoking has been shown to reduce the risk of lung cancer in exposed workers.

Asbestos

Epidemiology. The first data demonstrating a role for smoking in the causation of occupational cancer came from studies of asbestos workers. In 1968 Selikoff and co-workers (Selikoff et al., 1968) found in a cohort of 370 asbestos insulation workers that 24 died of bronchogenic cancer. All of the deaths were in people who were regular cigarette smokers. None of the 87 workers who had not smoked but had been exposed to asbestos died of bronchogenic cancer, although several did develop asbestosis or mesothelioma. Relative risk for smoking asbestos workers compared to nonsmoking, nonasbestos exposed workers was estimated as 72.

In a later and larger study of 933 workers in a plant which produced amosite asbestos products, 60 lung cancers were found (Selikoff et al., 1980). Fifty-five of these cancers occurred among 430 workers who were cigarette smokers. The relative risk for combined asbestos and smoking was computed to be 80, compared to 10 for smoking alone and 5 for asbestos exposure alone. Further analysis of data from 12,051 asbestos insulation workers with 450 cancer deaths illustrates that most lung cancers occur in persons exposed to both asbestos and cigarette smoke (Table 3) (Hammond et al., 1979). Had there been no smoking, but the same asbestos exposure, the cancer rate would have been only 10% of that observed.

Similar results have been reported for other cohort studies examining risks of lung cancers related to asbestos exposure and cigarette smoking (Berry et al., 1972; Hillerdal et al., 1983; Pastorino et al., 1984). A few studies have not shown multiplicative effects, but analysis of all the data are most consistent with a multiplicative rather than an additive effect (Saracci, 1977).

Pathophysiology. Several possible mechanisms of interaction between asbestos and smoking have been proposed. Asbestos may act as a foreign body, resulting in chronic inflammation, cell injury and repair (Becklake, 1982). Smoking acting primarily as a tumor promoter might impair the capacity of cells to repair injury, leading

TABLE 3.   Attributable Risk of Death of Lung Cancer From Smoking
           and Asbestos Exposure

Total Deaths	1946
Lung Cancer Deaths	450
Deaths Attributable To:	
Cigarette Smoking Alone	94
Asbestos Exposure Alone	44
Smoking and Asbestos	303
Deaths Unrelated to Smoking or Asbestos	9

(Table modified from Selikoff, 1981)

instead to malignancy. Asbestos may also adsorb, concentrate, and
slowly release carcinogens from tobacco smoke (Thomson et al.,
1978).

Important questions relating to asbestos and smoking remain un-
answered. For example, are there critical times in exposure to one
or the other which results in highest risks of cancer? The latency
for lung cancer in asbestos workers is about 37 years (Hillerdal
et al., 1983). Although control of asbestos has improved considerably in recent years, many workers have large body levels of asbestos. How effective is smoking cessation in persons heavily exposed
to asbestos 20 years ago? The multiple step carcinogenesis model
strongly points toward smoking cessation as an intervention which
could potentially reduce the cancer risk at any stage prior to
development of cancer.

Uranium Ore and Metal Miners

Epidemiology. Archer and co-workers first considered the role of
cigarette smoking in the development of cancer in uranium ore miners
(Archer et al., 1973). In their cohort, 39 workers died of lung
cancer. Comparing data from miners in that geographical location,
they estimated a relative risk of about 7 for lung cancer in uranium
miners without smoking, a relative risk of 4-8 in smokers who were
not miners, and a relative risk of 40 in miners who also smoked.
Smoking was also associated with a shorter induction latency period
in that nonsmokers and exsmoking uranium miners developed lung
cancer at an older age than current smokers.

A followup study was done on 4,000 uranium ore miners (Archer
et al., 1976). The population included white miners, who tended to
be smokers, and Indians who were nonsmokers or light smokers. The
incidence of bronchogenic cancer showed a relationship to cumulative
radiation exposure for smokers and nonsmokers. However, cigarette
smoking substantially amplified the lung cancer rates, particularly
at higher radiation exposure levels (Figure 2).

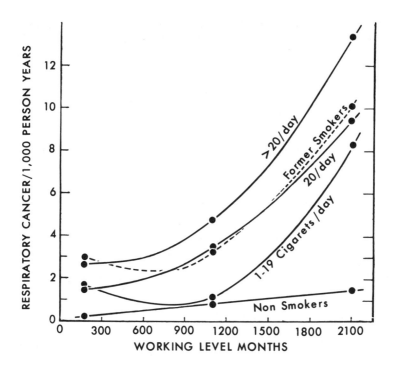

FIGURE 2. Dose-response relationship between cumulative radiation exposure (working level months) and respiratory cancer rate in uranium miners. Cigarette smoking amplifies the cancer rate, particularly at higher radiation exposure levels (Archer et al., 1976).

The multiplicative risk of cigarette smoking and radiation exposure in uranium miners was confirmed by a recent study of Whittemore and McMillan (1983). All three of the above studies indicate that smoking increases the rate of cancer fivefold or more in uranium miners.

Two studies, however, suggest that cancer risks in miners are lower in cigarette smokers. Axelson and Sundell (1978) conducted a case control study of lung cancer in Swedish zinc-lead miners, who were also exposed to radon daughters in the mines. In 29 lung cancer cases identified in one geographical area, most had worked in the mines and had a mortality ratio of 16.4 compared with those who were not miners. Nonsmokers tended to develop lung cancer more frequently than smokers; however, smokers developed cancer with a shorter average latency time and at a younger age.

Radford and Renard (1984) retrospectively studied a cohort of iron miners in another parish in Sweden. Fifty cancer deaths were identified. Nonsmokers had a risk ratio of 10 compared to 2.9 for

smokers. For the smokers, the absolute risks of occupation and
smoking appeared to be additive. In this study, time from initial
exposure to death was similar for smokers and nonsmokers.

In summary, three studies of United States uranium ore miners showed
multiplicative effects of smoking and occupational radiation exposure, while two studies of Swedish metal ore miners show additive
effects for smokers, but on average higher risks for nonsmokers.
Pathophysiologic considerations could explain both observations.

Pathophysiology. Uranium and other metal ores release radon gas,
which decays to daughters, two of which are alpha radiation emit-
ters. Presumably, the alpha radiation, when present in close proxi-
mity to bronchial cells, causes local damage and ultimately neoplasm. Radioactive gases may adsorb onto particles, which are then
inhaled and deposited within the lung. Cigarette smoke may be an
important source of particles for delivery of radiation to the lung
(Martell, 1983). Tobacco is also a source in itself of polonium 210
(Radford and Hunt, 1964). Therefore, smokers could have an additive
radiation risk in addition to that of other sources of radiation.
The carcinogenic effect of radiation could be promoted by tobacco
toxins, which would explain shorter onset and latency times.

The protective effect of cigarette smoking has been attributed to
mucous hypersecretion (Axelson and Sundell, 1978). Alpha radiation
has a short tissue penetration range. An increase in the thickness
of the mucous sheath in the airway of smokers, due to chronic bronchitis, could substantially reduce the effective radiation dose to
epithelial cells.

Arsenic (Copper Smelter) Workers

Epidemiology. Exposure to arsenic has been associated with an
increased risk of lung cancer in copper smelter workers, as well as
in pesticide manufacturers and vintners. In a case control study
with 76 lung cancer cases, Pershagen and co-workers (1981) found the
expected increase in lung cancer mortality risk for arsenic exposure
without smoking (relative risk 3.0), smoking without arsenic exposure (4.9) and multiplicative effects of both exposures (14.6). In
their analysis, it was estimated that 44% of cancers would have been
preventable if there was no arsenic exposure; 73% if there was no
cigarette smoking.

Welch and co-workers (1982) found in American smelter workers in
Montana that respiratory cancer rates were only slightly higher in
arsenic-exposed smokers compared to nonsmokers. The lung cancer
rates for the nonexposed smokers alone were not different from those
of nonsmokers, so the issue of multiplicative versus additive effects
could not be addressed.

An earlier study of copper smelter workers (Pinto et al., 1978),
which also reported an increased risk for arsenic exposure, showed
that smokers were at lower risk (2.9) for respiratory cancer than

nonsmokers (5.0). However, the number of cancer cases where smoking history was available was small (21) and there were only three cases in nonsmokers, so that the difference between smokers' and non-smokers' risk was not statistically significant.

Pathophysiology. The mechanism for carcinogenesis in copper smelter workers is not established. Arsenic is believed to be the most important toxin because of dose-related increases in cancer risk with increased arsenic exposure in several different occupations. Intratracheal administered arsenic can produce lung cancer in animals (Ivankovic et al., 1979). Arsenic may interfere with DNA repair (Rossman et al., 1975) and serve as a cocarcinogen. Other potential cancer-causing exposures of smelter workers include poly-aromatic hydrocarbons and other combustion products.

Chloromethyl Ethers: Does Smoking Protect Against Occupational Cancer?

Epidemiology. Chloromethyl ether (CME) and bischloromethyl ether, a contaminant, are known to be carcinogenic in animals and people. Chemical production workers exposed to CME experience a higher incidence of respiratory cancer, characterized by short latency and a small cell type histology. In a prospective study of 125 production workers followed for 10 years, there were 49 cases of respiratory cancers (Weiss, 1976). Cancer was related in a dose-related fashion to CME exposure, but inversely related to the number of cigarettes smoked. As expected, the prevalence of chronic lung disease was positively associated with CME exposure and cigarette smoking.

Pathophysiology. CME and bischloromethyl ether are alkylating chemicals which are believed to produce cancer by actions on DNA (Van Duuren et al., 1968). It has been hypothesized that the presence of bronchorrhea due to smoking-related chronic bronchitis dilutes, degrades and/or accelerates clearance of chloromethyl ethers. In support of the idea that smoking may protect against occupational lung cancer, Sterling (1983) reviewed studies indicating that (1) the dust content in lungs of smoking miners and millers contain less dust than nonsmoking miners; (2) smokers may clear some particles from the lung more quickly than nonsmokers; and (3) tobacco smoke exposure may reduce the incidence of respiratory cancer in animals inhaling radioactive radon daughters and uranium dust. An alterna-tive explanation for the "protective" effect of smoking is self-selection, such that workers heavily exposed to CME, which produces respiratory irritation and dyspnea, are less likely to smoke (Gold-smith, 1981). The reader is also referred to a comment by Higgins (1983) who criticizes the studies supporting the hypothesis that smoking has a protective effect against development of occupational lung cancer. He also cites animal studies showing that tobacco smoke can be cocarcinogenic with radon daughter exposure.

Lung Cancer in Workers: Occupation Versus Smoking

A number of studies showing increased lung cancer in workers in
particular occupations have been reviewed. There is convincing
evidence in asbestos workers and uranium ore miners that smoking
shifts the dose response curve for occupational exposure, resulting
in many more occupational cancers. Pastorino and co-workers (1984)
attempted to determine the relative importance of occupation and
smoking in causing lung cancer in a general population. They
studied all men in an industrial region of northern Italy. They
identified 204 cases of lung cancer and 351 controls in whom occupational histories could be obtained. Subjects were classified as
occupationally-exposed if they worked with any of the following
suspected respiratory carcinogens: asbestos, polycyclic aromatic
hydrocarbons, arsenic, nickel, chromium, bischloromethyl ether,
chloromethyl ether and vinyl chloride. About 80% of the cases and
the controls were cigarette smokers. The relative risk of lung
cancer was increased in workers with occupational exposure, and in

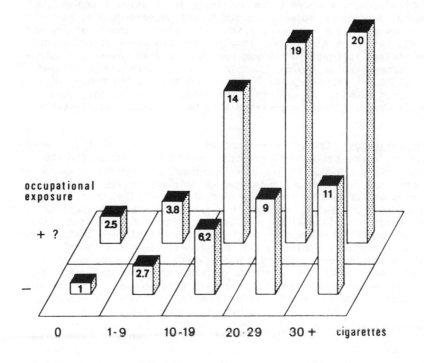

FIGURE 3. Risk of lung cancer in men in the Lombardy region of
Italy as a function of occupational exposure (to chemicals known to
cause lung cancer in humans) and daily cigarette consumption. Risks
of occupational exposure and smoking are multiplicative (Pastorino
et al., 1984).

a dose dependent manner for cigarette smokers (Figure 3). At all
smoking levels, the risk for exposed workers was twofold, indicating
a multiplicative effect. Overall, 33.0% (95% confidence interval,
19.1-46.9%) of cases were attributable to occupational exposure
(without modifying tobacco exposure) and 81.0% (95% CI, 68.8-93.2%)
to smoking (without modifying occupation). This study indicates
that in a general industrial worker population occupational exposure
to chemicals is a significant cause of cancer, but that most of it
would be prevented by smoking control. It also illustrates how an
association between occupational chemical exposure and lung cancer
risk might easily be missed where there is a high proportion of
cigarette smokers in the work force, unless very large worker populations are studied.

Factors Possibly Confounding the Relationship Between Smoking, Occupation and Cancer

Several factors may confound the smoking-occupational cancer interaction. Social class as a confounder has already been mentioned.
Blue collar, lower socioeconomic class workers are more likely to
smoke. Lower socioeconomic class may be associated with dietary
differences, greater consumption of alcohol, greater air pollution
in the home environment (due both to industrial pollution related to
geographical location of housing and higher probability of exposure
to tobacco smoke in the home). For further discussion of the potentially confounding effect of social class, the reader is referred to
Sterling (1978).

Diet may play a role in lung cancer risk. Several studies have
indicated an inverse relationship between vitamin A intake and the
development of lung cancer in smokers (Wald et al., 1980). Social
class and occupational factors could affect dietary tastes and
vitamin A intake. Smokers are more likely to drink heavily. Heavy
alcohol consumption predisposes to cancer of the nasopharynx, larynx
and esophagus, and these effects may be synergistic with those of
cigarette smoking (Schottenfeld, 1979).

Recent studies point to the possible role of radon gas in homes as
a potential cause of lung cancer (Harley, 1984). Radon gas may come
from the ground or from building construction materials. Higher
indoor radon concentrations are found in homes built of stone, brick
or plaster, in homes with basements and in homes built on high
radiation ground (alum shale zone) (Edling et al., 1984). Smoking,
as a marker of economic class, may be associated with geographical
location of homes and/or type of construction, and with indoor
radiation exposure. It has been suggested that cigarette smoke may
provide a nidus for passage of radon daughters into the lung
(Winters and DiFrenza, 1983).

Passive smoke exposure is a potentially confounding factor with respect to cancer rate in nonsmokers. This may be particularly important in a worker population, such as described in European cohorts
(Pastorino et al., 1984), where 80% of the workers are smokers.

PASSIVE SMOKING AND LUNG CANCER

Mainstream Versus Sidestream Cigarette Smoke

On average, 75% of the smoke generated in smoking a cigarette is
released into the environment (Hoegg, 1972; Schmeltz et al., 1975).
Sidestream smoke, that which is released into the environment, comes
from tobacco burned at a higher temperature with less oxygen compared to mainstream smoke. Concentrations of various toxic chemicals, including polyaromatic hydrocarbons, are higher in sidestream
compared to mainstream smoke. Sidestream smoke condensate is more
carcinogenic than mainstream smoke condensate (Schmeltz et al.,
1975). Irritant gases, like formaldehyde, ammonia and volatile
nitrosamines, are present in far greater concentration in sidestream
compared with mainstream smoke (Ayer and Yeager, 1982; Brunnemann
et al., 1977). Mainstream and sidestream smoke may also differ with
respect to particle size. Mainstream smoke particles are usually
0.1-0.2 microns, but as the smoke ages, which occurs in a smokey
room prior to inhalation by the nonsmoker, particles tend to coal-
esce, increasing size to about 0.6 microns (Guerin, 1980). The
latter are more likely to be deposited in the bronchioles rather
than in the alveoli. It has been suggested that inhalation of aged
smoke may increase the deposition of tar in the airways, which might
explain increased risk of cancer in passive smoking (Stock, 1982).
However, there is no experimental evidence at this time to support
the hypothesis.

Pathology and Pathogenesis of Lung Cancer in Smokers Versus Non-smokers

Smokers are more likely to develop Kreyberg I (squamous cell, oat
cell, small cell and large cell carcinoma) than Kreyberg II (primary
adenocarcinoma, bronchiolar and alveolar carcinoma) (Kabat and
Wynder, 1984). Nonsmokers are more likely to develop Kreyberg II.
For both smokers and nonsmokers, women are much more likely than men
to develop Kreyberg II compared to Kreyberg I cancers.

The difference in the pathology in lung cancer from primary smokers
and passive smokers suggests a different pathogenetic mechanism.
Possibly gaseous components of tobacco, which penetrate more deeply
into the periphery of the lung, are playing a causative role.

Evidence That Nonsmokers Inhale Cigarette Smoke

Several studies have provided evidence of tobacco smoke components
in the environment and in biological fluids of nonsmokers. Biochemical measures have included plasma and urinary nicotine and
cotinine (the latter a metabolite of nicotine) (Greenberg et al.,
1984; Russell, 1975; Wald et al., 1984); increased carboxyhemoglobin
(Russell et al., 1973) and plasma thiocyanate (Friedman et al.,
1983) (the latter a metabolite of cyanide, which is present in
tobacco smoke). Matsukura and co-workers (1984) showed equivalent

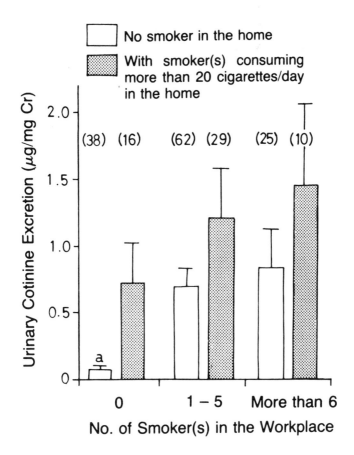

FIGURE 4.   Intake of environmental tobacco smoke by nonsmokers as
a function of number of smokers in the workplace. Cotinine is a
metabolite of nicotine. Urinary cotinine is an indicator of nicotine intake. Intake after workplace and home exposures are additive. Figures in parentheses indicate numbers of subjects in each
group. Bars indicate SEM. (Matsukura et al., 1984)

cotinine excretion in the urine in nonsmokers exposed to other
cigarette smokers in the home and in those exposed in the workplace.
Exposure in both places resulted in an increase in cotinine excretion (Figure 4). From urinary cotinine data, it is estimated that
nonsmokers may consume tobacco smoke equivalent to one to two cigarettes per day. There is overlap in the intake of heavily passively
exposed nonsmokers and light primary smokers.

General Hazards of Passive Smoking

Several authors have reviewed general issues of health hazards
associated with passive smoke exposure (Kabat and Wynder, 1984; Lee

1982; Repace. 1981; Weiss et al., 1983). In children there is a
higher incidence of respiratory infection in the first year of life
(Harlap and Davies, 1974), an increased prevalence of asthma
(Gortmaker et al., 1982) and some evidence of impaired pulmonary
function in children whose mothers smoke (Tager et al., 1983).
In adults, passive smoke exposure may aggravate angina pectoris
(Aronow, 1978) or asthma (Dahms et al., 1981), and may result in
mild impairment of small airway pulmonary function (White and Froeb,
1980), although the lifelong significance of the latter is still
unclear.

Lung Cancer and Passive Smoke Exposure

Three studies have reported a significantly increased risk of lung
cancer in nonsmokers who are passively exposed to cigarette smoke
(Table 4). The first report came from Hirayama (1981) who prospectively studied 142,800 women in Tokyo, of which 91,500 were nonsmoking wives. In a 14 year followup, he found 346 cases of lung
cancer, including 174 in the nonsmoking wives. The mortality ratio
for lung cancer in women who were smokers was 3.8. The risk of lung
cancer in nonsmoking wives with husbands who smoked was 1.6 if
husbands smoked less than 20, and 2.1 if husbands smoked more than
20 cigarettes per day. Since most men in Japan at the time of the
study smoked cigarettes, and most women did not, passive smoke
exposure appeared to be the most important cause of lung cancer in
Japanese women.

A number of criticisms of the study have been raised (Hammond and
Selikoff, 1981; Lee, 1982; Wynder and Goodman, 1983). These
included questions about statistical methods and comments about
cultural differences between Japanese and American wives, raising
the question of how relevant the results are for American women.
Subsequently, two small case control studies of lung cancer in women
reported significantly increased risk in those whose husbands smoked
(Correa et al., 1983; Trichopoulos et al., 1981). A fourth study,
the American Cancer Society study involving 469,000 nonsmokers

TABLE 4. Passive Smoking and Lung Cancer

Study	Type	Cases[†]	Relative Risk	
			Overall	Light/Heavy Exposure
Hirayama	P	174	1.8[*]	1.6[*] – 2.1[*]
Garfinkel	P	564	1.2	1.3 – 1.1
Trichopoulos	CC	38	2.7[*]	2.4[*] – 3.4[*]
Correa	CC	22	2.1[*]	1.2 – 3.5[*]

† - Female nonsmokers
* - P < 0.05
P = Prospective; CC = Case Control

studied prospectively, did not find a significantly increased risk (Garfinkel, 1981). A problem in all four studies is lack of verification of the extent of passive smoke exposure. The studies also suffer from the absence of occupational and other environmental tobacco smoke exposure data. This is a more significant problem in the American studies, because a larger percentage of American women, compared with Japanese or Greek women, work outside the home where they may be exposed to tobacco smoke or other chemical toxins.

Taking all the studies and their limitations, it appears that there is a small but real increase in lung cancer rate, with a relative risk of about 1.5, in passive smokers. Is the magnitude of that risk biologically plausible? There is a clear-cut dose response relationship between number of cigarettes smoked per day and the risk of lung cancer (Hammond and Horn, 1958). Assuming that passive smoke exposure is equivalent to smoking one cigarette per day, and assuming a linear dose response curve for cigarettes versus cancer risk, a relative risk of 1.5-2.0 is quite plausible.

Passive Smoking and Workplace Cancer

Data have been presented showing that workplace exposure to cigarette smoke can result in significant smoke intake, and that passive smoke exposure may be related to impaired respiratory function and an increased risk of lung cancer in nonsmokers. For nonsmokers sharing a work environment with cigarette smokers, the workplace must be considered hazardous independent of any specific industrial toxic exposure. This is particularly important when a high percentage of the workers smoke or when smokers and nonsmokers work in poorly ventilated areas.

Another concern is that passive smoke exposure acts synergistically, as does primary smoking, with industrial toxins to amplify the dose-response curve for those toxins. Although there is no empiric evidence to support this hypothesis at present, the possibility must be considered.

STRATEGIES TO CONTROL WORKPLACE SMOKING

Since (1) for primary cigarette smokers, smoking increases the risk of lung cancer following exposure to a given dose of certain occupational carcinogens and (2) cigarette smoke in the workplace environment probably presents an increased lung cancer risk to nonsmokers, smoking can no longer be viewed as purely a personal and private habit, the consequences of which are experienced only by the person who chooses to smoke. If the goal of an occupational health program is to prevent cancer (particularly in high risk occupations), the most effective way to do so is by control of cigarette smoking. The importance of controlling exposure to potentially carcinogenic industrial toxins is obvious, but total elimination of exposure is often impossible. An optimal employee health program should include simultaneous control of toxic exposures and smoking. A smoking control program should include both programs to encourage smoking cessation and environmental control measures to protect nonsmokers from tobacco smoke of their colleagues.

Smoking Cessation Strategies

Three general strategies are available for control of workplace smoking (Walsh, 1984). The first is development of programs to encourage employees to quit smoking. This includes physician counseling, educational activities, provision of smoking cessation programs in the workplace, or referral to outside cessation programs such as are available through the American Cancer Society or the American Lung Association (Danaher, 1980). Additionally, some businesses have offered various incentives for employees to quit. Despite the importance of smoking as a health problem, smoking control programs are offered only by about 8 to 15% of companies in various surveys (Walsh, 1984). Optimally, smoking cessation programs should be sponsored jointly by management and labor.

A second strategy is restricting or prohibiting smoking in the workplace. Many companies restrict smoking in certain work areas; however, the motives are usually related to protection of products or equipment, pleasing clients, or as required for control of explosion risks. Johns-Manville Corporation has restricted smoking in asbestos operations because of the potential synergistic effects between smoking and asbestos exposure. Such restriction seems to be the minimum that high risk industries should undertake.

The third strategy is not to hire cigarette smokers. Such extreme measures are unusual and fraught with legal difficulties. This approach is possible as evidenced by the Johns-Manville experience. When the risks of smoking and occupational exposure are clearly synergistic, such as with asbestos exposure and uranium mining, not hiring smokers seems quite sensible.

Control of Passive Smoke Exposure

The concentration of tobacco smoke in a room depends upon the size of the rooms, the number of smokers, the extent of ventilation and other factors such as the nature of wall surfaces (Hoegg, 1972; Repace and Lowrey, 1980). Ventilation with outside air and/or the use of high efficiency filtration systems substantially influences smoke concentrations, and is required at a minimum for workplace control of cigarette smoke. But even with good ventilation, such as with central air conditioning systems, substantial concentrations of CO and particulates are found in the workplace (Repace and Lowrey, 1980). So ventilation alone is not adequate.

Segregation of smokers and nonsmokers by space alone is partially effective, but primarily for particulates. In general, the greater the ratio of smoking to nonsmoking areas, the less effective the segregation (Repace, 1981). Studies of exposure to gaseous compounds like carbon monoxide in large rooms have shown no differences in smoking compared to nonsmoking sections (Olshansky, 1982). Placing physical barriers may be more effective, but the effectiveness depends on the amount of air flow between the segregated areas. However, in instances where it is not possible to place smokers and nonsmokers in separate rooms, barriers are better than nothing.

Prohibition of smoking in the work site is obviously the most effective way to reduce environmental smoke concentrations. Restricting workplace smoking so as to provide a smoke-free workplace for nonsmokers has been mandated legislatively in the State of Minnesota and recently in San Francisco. In both areas compliance appears to be good and enforcement has not been a major problem.

Air quality standards and permissible occupational exposure levels relevant to tobacco smoke components should be developed, monitored and enforced. This may be an important area of activity for the Occupational Safety and Health Administration (OSHA) (Kotin and Gaul, 1980).

Finally, where there is not adequate environmental control of cigarette smoke, nonsmoking workers should be advised of and given the opportunity to accept or reject the health risks of passive smoke exposure, as would be the case for workers in other hazardous environments.

CONCLUSIONS

Smoking in the workplace can be a cause of occupational cancer in smokers exposed to other occupational chemicals and probably in non-smokers exposed to tobacco smoke of other workers. Simultaneous control of workplace smoking and exposure to occupational toxins is necessary to minimize the likelihood of occupational cancer. Control of workplace smoking should be a combined effort of management and labor, and would be greatly benefited by support from OSHA.

ACKNOWLEDGEMENTS

Supported in part by Grants CA32389, DA02277 and DA01696 from the National Institutes of Health. I thank Dr. Charles Becker and Joseph LaDou for criticism and Ms. Kaye Welch for preparation of the manuscript.

REFERENCES

American Cancer Society: Cancer Facts & Figures. New York: American Cancer Society, 1983.

Archer VE, Gillam JD, Wagoner JK: Respiratory disease mortality among uranium miners. Ann NY Acad Sci 271:280-293, 1976.

Archer VE, Wagoner JK, Lundin FE: Uranium mining and cigarette smoking effects on man. J Occup Med 15:204-211, 1973.

Aronow WS: Effect of passive smoking on angina pectoris. N Engl J Med 299:21-24, 1978.

Auerbach O, Hammond EC, Garfinkel L: Changes in bronchial epithelium in relation to cigarette smoking, 1955-1960 vs. 1970-1977. N Engl J Med 300:381-386. 1979.

Axelson O, Sundell L: Mining, lung cancer and smoking. Scand J Work Environ & Health 4:46-52, 1978.

Ayer HE, Yeager DW: Irritants in cigarette smoke plumes. Am J Publ Health 72:1283-1285, 1985.

Becklake MR: Asbestos-related diseases of the lungs and pleura. Current clinical issues. Am Rev Respir Dis 126:187-194, 1982.

Berry G, Newhouse ML, Turok M: Combined effect of asbestos exposure and smoking on mortality from lung cancer in factory workers. Lancet 2:476-479, 1972.

Brunnemann KD, Yu L, Hoffmann D: Assessment of carcinogenic volatile N-nitrosamines in tobacco and in mainstream and sidestream smoke from cigarettes. Cancer Res 37:3218-3222, 1977.

Cairns J: The cancer problem. Sci American 233:64-78, 1975.

Correa P, Pickle LW, Fontham E, Lin Y, Haenszel W: Passive smoking and lung cancer. Lancet 2:595-597, 1983.

Covey LS, Wynder EL: Smoking habits and occupational status. J Occup Med 23:537-542, 1981.

Dahms TE, Bolin JF, Slavin RG: Passive smoking: Effects on bronchial asthma. Chest 80:530-534, 1981.

Danaher BG: Smoking cessation programs in occupational settings. Public Health Reports 95:149-157, 1980.

Doll R, Peto R: The causes of cancer: Quantitative estimates of avoidable risks of cancer in the United States today. J Natl Cancer Inst 66:1191-1308, 1981.

Edling C, Kling H, Axelson O: Radon in homes - A possible cause of lung cancer. Scand J Work Environ Health 10:25-34, 1984.

Friedman GD, Petitti DB, Bawol RD: Prevalence and correlates of passive smoking. Am J Publ Health 73:401-405, 1983.

Garfinkel L: Time trends in lung cancer mortality among nonsmokers and a note on passive smoking. J Natl Cancer Inst 66:1061-1066, 1981.

Goldsmith JR: Cigarette smoking, lung cancer and CME - A clarification (Letter). J Occup Med 23:77-78, 1981.

Gortmaker SL, Walker DK, Jacobs FH, Ruch-Ross H: Parental smoking and the risk of childhood asthma. Am J Publ Health 72:574-579, 1982.

Greenberg RA, Haley NJ, Etzel RA, Loda FA: Measuring the exposure of infants to tobacco smoking: Nicotine and cotinine in urine and saliva. N Engl J Med 310:1075-1078, 1984.

Guerin MR: Chemical composition of cigarette smoke. In: Banbury Report 3. A Safe Cigarette?, edited by GB Gori, FG Bock, pp. 191-204. Cold Spring Harbor Laboratory, 1980.

Hammond EC, Horn D: Smoking and death rates - Report on forty-four months of follow-up of 187,783 men. J Am Med Assn 166:1294-1308, 1958.

Hammond EC, Selikoff IJ: Passive smoking and lung cancer with comments on two new papers. Environ Res 24:444-452, 1981.

Hammond EC, Selikoff IJ, Seidman H: Asbestos exposure, cigarette smoking and death rates. Ann NY Acad Sci 330:473-490, 1979.

Harlap S, Davies AM: Infant admissions to hospital and maternal smoking. Lancet 1:529-532, 1974.

Harley NH: Radon and lung cancer in mines and homes. N Engl J Med 310:1525-1527, 1984.

Harris JE: Cigarette smoking among successive birth cohorts on men and women in the United States during 1900-1980. J Natl Cancer Inst 71:473-479, 1983.

Higgins ITT: Commentary on "possible effects on occupational lung cancer from smoking related changes in the mucus content of the lung." J Chron Dis 36:677-680, 1983.

Hillerdal G, Karlen E, Aberg T: Tobacco consumption and asbestos exposure in patients with lung cancer: A three year prospective study. Brit J Indus Med 40:380-383, 1983.

Hirayama T: Nonsmoking wives of heavy smokers have a higher risk of lung cancer: A study from Japan. Brit Med J 282:183-185, 1981.

Hoegg UR: Cigarette smoke in closed spaces. Environ Health Perspect 2:117-127, 1972.

Hoffmann D, Schmeltz I, Hecht SS, Wynder EL: Tobacco carcinogenesis. In: Polycyclic Hydrocarbons and Cancer, Vol. 1, edited by H Gelboin. PO Tso, pp. 119-130. New York: Academic Press, 1978.

Ivankovic S, Eisenbrand G, Preussmann R: Lung carcinoma induction in BD rats after single intratracheal instillation of an arsenic-containing pesticide mixture formerly used in vineyards. Int J Cancer 24:786-789, 1979.

Kabat GC, Wynder EL: Lung cancer in nonsmokers. Cancer 53:1214-1221, 1984.

Kilburn KH: Particles causing lung disease. Environ Health Perspec 55:97-109, 1984.

Kotin P, Gaul LA: Smoking in the workplace: A hazard ignored. Am J Publ Health 70:575-576, 1980.

Lee PN: Passive smoking. Food Chem Toxicol 20:223-229, 1982.

Martell EA: Alpha-radiation dose at bronchial bifurcations of smokers from indoor exposure to radon progeny. Proc Natl Acad Sci USA 80:1285-1289, 1983.

Matsukura S, Taminato T, Kitano N, Seino Y, Hamada H, Uchihashi M, Nakajima H, Hirata Y: Effects of environmental tobacco smoke on urinary cotinine excretion in nonsmokers. N Engl J Med 311:828-832, 1984.

Olshansky SJ: Is smoker/nonsmoker segregation effective in reducing passive inhalation among nonsmokers? Am J Publ Health 72:737-739, 1982.

Pastorino U, Berrino F, Gervasio A, Pesenti V, Riboli E, Crosignani P: Proportion of lung cancers due to occupational exposure. Int J Cancer 33:231-237, 1984.

Pershagen G, Wall S, Taube A, Linnman L: On the interaction between occupational arsenic exposure and smoking and its relationship to lung cancer. Scand J Work Environ Health 7:302-309, 1981.

Pinto SS, Henderson V, Enterline PE: Mortality experience of arsenic-exposed workers. Arch Environ Health 33:325-331, 1978.

Radford EP, Hunt VR: Polonium-210: A volatile radioelement in cigarettes. Science 143:247-249, 1964.

Radford EP, Renard KGS: Lung cancer in Swedish iron miners exposed to low doses of radon daughters. N Engl J Med 310:1485-1494, 1984.

Repace JL: The problem of passive smoking. Bull NY Acad Med 57:936-946, 1981.

Repace JL, Lowrey AH: Indoor air pollution, tobacco smoke, and public health. Science 208:464-472, 1980.

Rossmann T, Meyn MS, Troll W: Effects of sodium arsenite in the survival of UV-irradiated Escherichia coli: Inhalation of a recA-dependent function. Mutat Res 38:157-162, 1975.

Russell MAH, Cole PV, Brown E: Absorption by nonsmokers of carbon monoxide from room air polluted by tobacco smoke. Lancet 1:576-579, 1973.

Russell MAH, Feyerabend C: Blood and urinary nicotine in non-smokers. Lancet 1:179-181, 1975.

Sachs DPL: Smoking habits of pulmonary physicians (Letter). N Engl J Med 309:799, 1983.

Saracci R: Asbestos and lung cancer: An analysis of the epidemiological evidence on the asbestos-smoking interaction. Int J Cancer 20:323-331, 1977.

Schmeltz I, Hoffmann D, Wynder EL: The influence of tobacco smoke on indoor atmospheres. I. An overview. Preventive Med 4:66-82, 1975.

Schottenfeld D: Alcohol as a cofactor in the etiology of cancer. Cancer 43:1962-1966, 1979.

Selikoff IJ: Two comments on smoking and the workplace (Letter). Am J Publ Health 71:92, 1981.

Selikoff IJ, Hammond EC, Churg J: Asbestos exposure, smoking, and neoplasia. J Amer Med Assn 204:104-110, 1968.

Selikoff IJ, Seidman H, Hammond EC: Mortality effects of cigarette smoking among amosite asbestos factory workers. J Natl Cancer Inst 65:507-513, 1980.

Sterling TD: Does smoking kill workers or working kill smokers? or The mutual relationship between smoking, occupation, and respiratory disease. Int J Health Serv 8:437-452, 1978.

Sterling TD: Possible effects on occupational lung cancer from smoking related changes in the mucus content of the lung. J Chron Dis 10:669-676, 1983.

Sterling TD, Weinkam JJ: Smoking characteristics by type of employment. J Occup Med 18:743-754, 1976.

Stock SL: Passive smoking and lung cancer (Letter). Lancet 1:1014-1015, 1982.

Surgeon General of US: Health consequences of smoking: Cancer. Rockville, MD: Dept. of Health and Human Services, 1982.

Tager IB, Weiss ST, Munoz A, Rosner B, Speizer FE: Longitudinal study of the effects of maternal smoking on pulmonary function in children. N Engl J Med 309:699-703, 1983.

Thomson R, Kilroe-Smith TA, Webster I: The effect of asbestos-associated metal ions on the binding of benzo(a)pyrene to macromolecules In vitro. Environ Res 15:309, 1978.

Trichopoulos D, Kalandidi A, Sparros L, MacMahon B: Lung cancer and passive smoking. Int J Cancer 27:1-4, 1981.

Van Duuren BL, Goldschmidt BM, Katz C, Langseth L, Mercado G, Sivak A: Alpha-haloethers: A new type of alkylating carcinogen. Arch Environ Health 16:472-476, 1968.

Wald NJ, Boreham J, Bailey A, Ritchie C, Haddow JE, Knight G: Urinary cotinine as marker of breathing other people's tobacco smoke. Lancet 1:230-231, 1984.

Wald N, Idle M, Boreham J, Bailey A: Low serum vitamin A and subsequent risk of cancer. Lancet 3:813-815, 1980.

Walsh DC: Corporate smoking policies: A review and an analysis. J Occup Med 26:17-22, 1984.

Weiss ST, Tager IB, Speizer FE: Passive smoking: Its relationship to respiratory symptoms, pulmonary function and nonspecific bronchial responsiveness. Chest 84:651, 1983.

Weiss W: Chloromethyl ethers, cigarettes, cough and cancer. J Occup Med 18:194-199, 1976.

Welch K, Higgins I, Oh M, Burchfiel C: Arsenic exposure, smoking and respiratory cancer in copper smelter workers. Arch Envir Health 37:325-335, 1982.

White JR, Froeb HF: Small-airways dysfunction in nonsmokers chronically exposed to tobacco smoke. N Engl J Med 302:720-723, 1980.

Whittemore AS, McMillan A: Lung cancer mortality among U.S. uranium miners: A reappraisal. J Natl Cancer Inst 71:489-499, 1983.

Winters TH, DiFrenza J: Radioactivity and lung cancer in active and passive smokers. Chest 84:653-654, 1983.

Wynder EL, Goodman WT: Smoking and lung cancer: Some unresolved issues. Epid Rev 5:177-207, 1983.

14

Overview of the Ronald E. Talcott Symposium: Quinones as Mutagens, Carcinogens, and Anticancer Agents

MARTYN T. SMITH

Dr. Ronald Talcott and I shared a mutual interest in the metabolism and toxicity of quinones. Just prior to his untimely death, Ron was actively pursuing research on the metabolism and toxicity of various substituted naphthoquinones with the aim of selectively killing human brain tumor cells. A review of this work was presented at the symposium by Dr. Mitchell Berger, a clinical colleague of Ron's, and will be discussed later in this brief summary. Quinones are diketones derived from aromatic compounds so that the two carbonyl groups may be in the same or different rings. They are widely distributed in nature where they are centrally involved in many electron transport and biosynthetic processes. Many natural quinone pigments are used as dyes and the therapeutic qualities of certain quinones have been investigated in detail[1]. Quinones form an important toxic defense system for many insects and anthropods[2] and are common environmental pollutants[3,4]. Perhaps more importantly, quinone metabolites have been proposed as being involved in the toxicity and carcinogenicity of many different chemicals, including benzene, benzo(a)pyrene and diethylstilbesterol. The first three papers presented at the symposium by Drs. Irons, Lesko and Liehr addressed the role of quinone metabolites in the toxic effects of these three chemicals.

Dr. Richard Irons of the Chemical Industry Institute of Toxicology, Research Triangle Park, gave an overview of quinones as toxic metabolites of benzene. Although the metabolism of benzene is complex[5], the quinone metabolites of benzene have proven to be toxic to bone marrow and lymphoid cells both in vivo and in vitro. p-Benzoquinone, for example, is a remarkably potent inhibitor of mitogen-induced lymphocyte mitogenesis and Dr. Irons' studies point to the notion that it does this by disrupting microtubule-dependent cell functions through its arylation of tubulin thiol groups. Gaining an understanding of exactly which toxic metabolite(s) is responsible for benzene's toxic effects on the bone marrow would greatly improve our ability to predict the risk to workers occupationally exposed to benzene.

Benzo(a)pyrene (BP) is, of course, a classic carcinogen and is metabolized to a number of highly reactive intermediates, including a
number of diol epoxides. One of these, the anti-isomer of
BP-7,8-dihydrodiol-9,10-epoxide, is presumed to be the ultimate carcinogenic metabolite of BP. BP is, however, also metabolised to
three isomeric quinones. These three quinones can account for up to
50% of the BP metabolites formed and have recently been shown to be
mutagenic in the new Salmonella tester strain TA104 through their
ability to generate active oxygen species[6]. Dr. Stephen Lesko of
Johns Hopkins University School of Hygiene and Public Health presented a detailed review of the toxic properties of these BP quinones and discussed their possible role in both promoting and initiating BP carcinogenesis.

Diethylstilbesterol (DES) is a known animal and human carcinogen.
The mechanism by which DES produces tumors is controversial. Dr.
Joachim Liehr of the University of Texas Medical School at Houston
presented work which showed that the estrogenicity of estradiols,
including DES, can be separated from their carcinogenicity. Thus,
estrogens of high hormonal potency are not necessarily carcinogens.
A role for DES quinone in DES carcinogenesis has been repeatedly
postulated but its improved synthesis and description of its spec-
tral properties by Dr. Liehr's group has enabled them to demonstrate
its formation by peroxidase enzymes in vitro[7]. Dr. Liehr also presented further work at the symposium which supported a role for DES
quinone in DES carcinogenesis.

The second part of the symposium consisted of two talks on the origins of human brain tumors and their possible therapy with quinones.
Dr. Andrew Moss of the University of California, San Francisco,
discussed the epidemiological evidence for an occupational risk of
brain cancer which has been reported in four industries, most
notably the petrochemical industry. Vinyl chloride remains, however, the only known occupational CNS carcinogen and Dr. Moss discussed the link between human brain tumors and this chemical in detail.

Dr. Mitchell Berger of the Brain Tumor Research Center, University
of California, San Francisco, described the work he, Dr. Talcott,
Dr. Marilyn Silva and others had done regarding the possible therapy of human brain tumors with halogen-substituted 1,4-naphthoqui-
nones, first described by Lin et al.[8] as potential bioreductive alkylating agents. Dr. Berger described how brain tumor cells derived from malignant gliomas contain very high levels of the enzyme
DT-diaphorase. This enzyme activates the above halogenated quinones to highly reactive quinone methides, which are highly toxic
to brain tumor cells and being as they are small and very lipo-
philic they easily cross the blood barrier, making them potentially
useful as therapeutic drugs for human brain tumors.

Quinones may therefore be either toxic or therapeutic and their prevalence makes them an important group to study. This symposium
will be published as a series of papers by each speaker in a future
edition of the Journal of Toxicology and Environmental Health.

ACKNOWLEDGEMENT

This symposium was supported, in part, by a grant from the University of California Cancer Research Coordinating Committee.

REFERENCES

1. Moore HW, Czerniak R: Naturally occuring quinones as potential bioreductive alkylating agents. Med Res Revs 1:249-280, 1981.

2. Vukasovic P, Stojanovic T, Kosovac V: Les insectes s'attaquant aux graines de tournesol (Helianthe, Helianthes annus L.) en Yugoslavie. J Stored Prod Res 2:69-73, 1966.

3. Fox MA, Olive S: Photooxidation of anthracene on atmospheric particulate matter. Science 205:582-583, 1979.

4. Scheutzle D: Sampling of vehicle emissions for chemical analysis and biological testing. Environ Health Perspect 47:65-80, 1983.

5. Irons RD, Dent JG, Baker TS, Rickert DE: Benzene is metabolised and covalently bound in bone marrow in situ. Chem-Biol Interact 30:241-245, 1980.

6. Chesis PL, Levin DE, Smith MT, Ernster L, Ames BN: Mutagenicity of quinones: Pathways of metabolic activation and detoxification. Proc Natl Acad Sci 81:1696-1700, 1984.

7. Liehr JG, DaGue BB, Ballatore AM, Henkin J: Diethylstibesterol (DES) quinone: A reactive intermediate in DES metabolism. Biochem Pharmacol 32:3711-3718, 1983.

8. Lin AJ, Pardini RS, Cosby LA, Lillis BJ, Shansky CW, Sartorelli AC: Potential bioreductive alkylating agents. 2. Antitumor effects and biochemical studies of naphthoquinone derivatives. J Med Chem 16:1268-1271, 1973.

15

Controversies in the Assessment of Carcinogenic Risk of Formaldehyde

JON ROSENBERG

INTRODUCTION

Volatile, colorless, pungent gas
Reactive: polymerizes with self
condenses with self
condenses to form methyloyl or methylene derivatives
reacts with HCl to form bis(chloromethyl) ether

World production over 10 billion pounds
U.S. production over 6 billion pounds
60% for plactics and resins
22% for production of intermediates
18% for miscellaneous uses

Incomplete combustion of hydrocarbons
666 million pounds U.S. from mobile engines
13.1 million pounds U.S. from municipal incinerators
cigarette smoke 40-100 ppm (0.4 mg/day)

Occupational Exposure
U.S. 8,000 workers production, 1.5 million total
Embalming 0.1-0.4 ppm/Resin manufacture 1-30 ppm
3.5%   3 ppm, 12%   1 ppm, 88%   0.5 ppm (Siegal et al, 1983)

OCCUPATIONAL EXPOSURE LIMITS

U.S.	PPM	Yr. Est.
OSHA	3 TWA	1973
NIOSH	1 Ceiling	1976
ACGIH	2 Ceiling	1980
	(1 A2	1984)
Belgium	2 Ceiling	1978
Finland	2 Ceiling	1975
F.R. Germany	1 TWA	1979
Italy	1 TWA	1978

U.S.	PPM	Yr. Est.
Sweden	2 Ceiling	1978
Switzerland	1 TWA	1978

Environmental Exposure
U.S. Mobile Homes 10 million people 0.03-2.5 ppm
U.S. Foam Insulation 1 million people 0.01-5 ppm
U.S. Non-foam Insulation 98 million people 0.01-0.1 ppm

A. Carcinogenicity in Animals

CIIT Study (CIIT, 1981 and Swenberg et al, 1980).

Rat: Groups of 120 male and female Fischer 344 rats were exposed
to 0,2,5.6 or 14.3 ppm for 6 hrs/day, 5 days/week for up to 24
months, followed by a 6 month observation period. Some animals
were sacrified at intervals of 6 months. Increases in squamous-
cell carcinoma of the nasal cavity were observed at 14.3 ppm in
male (51 of 117) and female (52 of 115) rats, compared to 5.6 ppm
(1 of 119 and 1 of 116) and 2.0 and 0 (none). No other neoplasm
was increased significantly.

Mouse: B6C3F Mice, as above. Squamous-cell carcinomas in nasal
cavities occurred in 2 male mice at 14.3 ppm, no others; not
statistically significant.

New York University Study (Albert et al, 1982)

Rat: Groups of 100 male Sprague-Dawley rats were exposed to 14
ppm formaldehyde and 10 ppm hydrogen chloride gas, 10 ppm hydrogen
chloride gas alone or air, for 6 hours/day, 5 days/week for life.
Squamous-cell carcinoma of the nasal cavity occurred in at 14.3
ppm formaldehyde alone. In a preliminary report, after 19.4 mo.
10/100 rats at 14 ppm formaldehyde above had squamous-cell nasal
cancer, compared to 12/100 and 6/100 in the 2 combined-exposure
groups, and 0/100 in HCl and air exposed groups. In an earlier
study, 25/99 rats had squamous-cell nasal cancer after combined
14 ppm formaldehyde and 10 ppm hydrogen chloride exposure for life.

B. Effective Dose Delivery In Animals

The tumors observed in the above animal studies are all at the
first point of contact with formaldehyde. Formaldehyde is highly
water soluble. Studies with radiolabeled formaldehyde have shown
that most of an inhaled dose in rats is abosrbed in the upper
respiratory tract, with highest concentrations in the anterior
nasal mucosa (Heck et al, 1983). This distribution of formaldehyde correlates well with the observed lesions, including carcinomas, in rodents. Variables affecting the dose delivered to the
nasal mucosa include formaldehyde concentration, the minute volume
(respiratory rate x tidal volume) and nasal surface area. These
variables were compared for rat and mouse to hypothesize an explanation for the observed species differences in sensitivity to form-

aldehyde. (Barrow et al, 1983). Rats have a larger surface area
than mice (13.44 vs 2.89 cm) and lower respiratory rates before
exposure to formaldehyde. However, mice have a much smaller tidal
volume before exposure, and are more sensitive to the sensory irritation from formaldehyde at high levels of exposure (1 ppm),
which results in further decreases in tidal volume. Thus, the
theoretical dose of formaldehyde of the nasal mucosa during 15 ppm
exposure for the rat is twice that for the mouse. This may contribute to interspecies differences, although differences in
metabolism mucociliary clearance, nasal cavity blood flow, nasal
endothelial cell type distribution and others may also play
important roles.

C. Effective Dose Delivery in Humans

Rodents are obligatory nose breathers, humans breathe through the
nose and mouth. The dose delivered to the human nasal mucosa at
the same levels of exposure may be less than the rodent. The dose
delivered to the oral cavity, trachea and possibly the lungs may be
more. The relevance of this to carcinogenic risk cannot be determined at the present time.

D. Cytotoxicity of Formaldehyde

Formaldehyde is cytotoxic, an effect which is more dependent upon
concentration than cumulative dose. A number of histopathologic
changes in the nasal cavities of rat and mice attribute to cytotoxic or irritant effects were observed in the CIIT study (CIIT,
1981 and Swenberg et al, 1980). These effects, which included
rhinitis, epithelial dysplasia, squamous metaplasia, and squamous
or epithelial hyperplasia, were generally dose dependent, greater
in rats than mice, greater in anterior than posterior nasal cavity
sections, and showed apparent regression after cessation of
exposure for all sections except in the anterior cavities of high
exposure rats. Persistent cytotoxic changes were therefore
correlated with the formation of neoplastic lesions, but with some
exceptions.

E. Effect of Cytotoxicity on Cell Turnover

The significance of cytotoxicity lies in the hypothesis, that,
since cytotoxicity is usually associated with increases in cell
turnover (to replace losses), and increases in cell turnover are
accompanied by increased replication of DNA, increased errors in
replication might occur, and therefore mutation and carcinogenesis.
However, this process of carcinogenesis, termed "epigenetic", would
result in a dose-response relationship that would display a threshold at levels of exposure below the threshold for cytotoxicity.
Most "epigenetic" carcinogens are identified by a lack of genotoxicity in short-term tests. Formaldehyde exposure is associated
with increases in cell turnover, measured by radiolabeled thymidine
autoradiography, in rats exposed to 6 and 15 ppm but not 0.5 or
2.90 ppm for 3 days, and in mice exposed to 15 ppm but not the
lower levels. (Swenberg et al, 1983 a,b). The relationship of
this to carcinogenic risk remains speculative, particularly in view

of the genotoxicity of formaldehyde (see below).

F. Genotoxicity of Formaldehyde

Formaldehyde Institute/Litton Bionetics Battery (Brusick, 1983)

Test	Response	MFC	Comments
Ames Salmonella Reverse Mutation	-	Up to 1000ug	NTP + with pre-incubation
Mouse Lymphoma	+	1.9ug/ml(S9) 7.5ug/ml(no S9)	Dose-response
CHO SCE	+	0.5ug/ml(S9) 1.0ug/ml(no S9)	No dose-response
CHO Aberrvation	-	4.0ug/ml	Alk agents not clastogenic
Cell Transformation (Balb/c3T3)	+	0.5-2.5ug/ml	Dose-response
Mouse SCE In Vivo	+Female	?12,25 ppm	Prelim. results

IARC (1982) Review

Test	Response	Comments
E coli Mutation	+	DNA repair enz def spec more sens
S. cerevisiae Mutation	+	DNA repair enz def spec more sens
CHO SCE	+	
Human lymphocyte SCE	+	
HeLa Cell UDS	+	
Mouse 4210 DNA-protein crosslinks	+	Mutation assays above indicate DNA protein crosslinks
Drosophila	+ -	Depending on mode of administration

Summary (IARC, 1982): Formaldehyde causes DNA damage in bacteria, yeast and mammalian cells, is mutagenic to bacteria, yeasts and Drosophilia, but not to the silkworm nor to mammalian cells in culture, causes chromosomal aberrations in mammalians cells, plants and the spermatocytes of grasshoppers and fruit flies, and has been reported to be both positive and negative for dominant lethal mutations in mice.

Comment: The genotoxicity of formaldehyde has been described some as "weak," on the basis of both potency and occurrence of negative tests. The activity of formaldehyde in the above positive controls, such as ethylmethane sulfonate and dimethylnitrosamine.

However, those tests that were negative are not necessarily indicative of weak activity, but rather of specificity of activity.

G. Risk Assessment

ISSUES

Epigenetic vs. genetic

It has been hypothesized that formaldehyde promotes its own carcinogencity through its cytotoxic effects at high levels of exposure, thus resulting in a non-linear dose response-curve, as observed in rats, if not an actual threshold of non-response (Swenberg et al, 1983b).

Cytotoxicity and significance of metaplasia

Species difference

Effective dose

Mucociliary clearance and other defenses

Metabolism and significant of formaldehyde in normal cells

It has been stated that "intuitively" the efforts of low levels of formaldehyde must be limited due to its occurrence as a normal endogenous metabolic product (Gibson, 1982). However, the process that limits the effects of endogenously formed formaldehyde may not be effective against exogenous formaldehyde.

Extrapolation to humans

Doses for 1/1 million risk of cancer in rats, adjusted for numbers of animals at risk (from Gibson, 1982).

Model	Dose (ppm)
Probit	2.14
Multihit	1.52
Logit	0.89
Weibull	0.76
Multistage	0.65
Linear	0.00059

Direct extrapolation to workers by the multistage model yields a risk of 620/100,000 (maximum liklihood) or 930/100,000 (upper 95% confidence limit) at 3 ppm (6h/d, 5d/w, lifetime) (Siegel et al, 1983). Even if the risk is assured to be 100-times less, this still represents a generally unacceptable level of risk.

References

Albert, RE, Sellakumar, AR, Laskin, S et al: Gaseous formaldehyde
and hydrogen chloride induction of nasal cancer in the rat. JNCI
68:597-603, 1982.

Barrow, CS, Steinhagan, WH and Chang, JCF: Formaldehyde sensory
irritation. Chapter 3 in Gibson (ed), 1983.

Brusick, DJ: Genetic and transforming activity of formaldehyde.
Chapter 8 in Gibson (ed), 1983.

Chemical Industry Institution of Technology (CIIT): Final Report
on a Chronic Inhalation Toxicology Study in Rats and Mice Exposed
to Formaldehyde. Conducted by Battelle Laboratory, Columbus, Ohio,
for CIIT, 1981.

Gibson, JE (ed): Formaldehyde Toxicity. Hemisphere, New York, 1983.

Gibson, JE: Risk assessment using a combination of testing and
research results. Chapter 26 in Gibson (ed), 1983.

International Agency for Research on Cancer (IARC). Monographs on
the evaluation of the carcinogenicity of chemicals to humans: some
industrial chemicals and dyestuffs. Volume 29:345-349, 1982.

Siegel, DM, Frankos, VH and Schneiderman, MA: Formaldehyde risk
assessment for occupationally exposed workers. Reg Toxicol
Pharmacol 3:355-371, 1983.

Swenberg JA, Kerns, WD, Mitchell, RI et al: Induction of squamous
cell carcinomas or the rat nasal cavity by inhalation exposure to
formaldehyde vapor. Cancer Res 40:3398-3402, 1980.

Swenberg JA, Barrow, CS, Bareiko, CJ et al: Non-linear biological
responses to formaldehyde and their implications for carcinogenicity risk assessment. Carcinogenesis 4:945-952, 1983 (a).

Swenberg, JA , Gross, EA, Martin, J and Popp, JA: Mechanisms of
formaldehyde toxicity. Chapter 12 in Gibson (ed), 1983(b).

Index